D1435355

The Complete Home Medical Guide for Dogs

STEPHEN SCHNECK AND DR. NIGEL NORRIS

The Complete Home Medical Guide for Dogs

STEIN AND DAY/ *Publishers*/ New York

First published in 1976
Copyright © 1976 by Stephen Schneck
All rights reserved
Designed by David Miller
Printed in United States of America
Stein and Day/*Publishers*/ Scarborough House,
Briarcliff Manor, N.Y. 10510

SECOND PRINTING 1976

Library of Congress Cataloging in Publication Data

Schneck, Stephen, 1933-
    The complete home medical guide for dogs.

    1. Dogs—Diseases. I. Norris, Nigel, joint author.
II. Title.
SF991.S3155   636.7'08'96024   74-31110
ISBN 0-8128-1798-2

Introduction

One of the many problems facing veterinaries is how to explain, in non-technical language, what is wrong with a pet animal so that the owner can understand and, if possible, help the healing process. The layman can only be expected to have a superficial knowledge of anatomy and physiology, and the rapid advances in diagnosis and treatment in recent years have made the gulf between professional advisor and client even wider.

Veterinarians in small-animal practice soon gain experience in explaining, as simply as possible, what may be a very complex condition. Nevertheless, most of us have felt the need for an up-to-date book compiled especially for the pet owner.

The Complete Home Medical Guide for Dogs, written by a pet owner in collaboration with a practicing veterinarian, neatly fills this gap. Factually correct, the information is presented in clear everyday language which will give useful guidance to even the most inexperienced owner with little or no knowledge of biology.

In many parts of the world, a dog or cat owner may be far from the nearest veterinary, and though in some countries flying doctor services are available, the "flying vet" is, as yet, a luxury pet owners cannot afford. In these remote areas antibiotics and other medicines are available, but they are of little use without some knowledge and advice on how to use them. In the United Kingdom and the United States, as well as in many other countries, antibiotics, etc. are (quite rightly) sold only on prescription. There are, however, many simple and effective remedies which can be used before professional advice is sought, or when it is not possible to get immediate treatment from a vet. This book helps the owner to cope with both situations and also gives the basic rules for prompt and effective first-aid in emergencies.

Veterinarians, of course, are most concerned that people should look after their pets in a responsible way. This means caring for the health and welfare of the animal and being alert for any changes which may be signs of impending illness. *The Complete Home Medical Guide for Dogs* should be of considerable help in furthering this aim and will, I am sure, be welcomed by both pet owners and veterinarians.

Henry Carter, MRCVS
Past President
British Small Animal Veterinary Association

How to Use
This Book

Successful home medical treatment is based on the ability to make the correct medical diagnosis. A sick or injured animal exhibits certain symptoms. These symptoms are signs which, properly observed, lead to an intelligent and informed diagnosis.

This book has been specially designed to help the responsible pet owner make this diagnosis.

Every symptom likely to be exhibited by a sick or injured animal is listed in the Index. There is also a Table of Contents which lists the entries according to the parts of the body affected. If, for example, the animal is suffering from ear mites (Otodectic Mange) treatment for this condition will be found by referring to the Table of Contents under problems of Head and Neck. However, if the pet owner does not know that excessive scratching of the ear, shaking of the head, a discharge from the ear, or waxy, brown crusts in the ear suggests ear mites, any of these symptoms can be found in the Index and the reader will be referred to the appropriate entry. If, as in this instance, home treatment is possible, this treatment will be described in the entry. When home treatment is not recommended, the entry will inform the reader.

Of course it is not always possible to make accurate diagnoses solely on the basis of simple observation. Many diseases can be diagnosed only by a veterinary with laboratory facilities.

No book, however informative, can substitute for professional treatment. What this book can do, is to inform the pet owner when a vet's services are necessary, what constitutes an emergency, and, in many cases, serve as a temporary paramedical aid when a vet is not immediately available.

Contents

2. PROBLEMS OF THE HEAD AND NECK

3. PROBLEMS OF THE SKIN AND HAIR

4. PROBLEMS OF THE CHEST

5. PROBLEMS OF THE ABDOMEN

6. PROBLEMS OF THE ANORECTAL REGION

7. PROBLEMS OF THE URINARY SYSTEM

8. PROBLEMS OF THE EXTREMITIES

9. PROBLEMS OF THE BACK

10. PROBLEMS AFFECTING THE WHOLE BODY

11. PROBLEMS OF FEMALE DOGS ONLY

12. POISONING

The Complete
Home
Medical Guide
for Dogs

1

General
Dog Care

Analgesics

Analgesics are used to relieve pain. While there are many pain relievers available, we recommend simple 5-grain aspirin tablets.

When to administer: When the dog is in obvious pain or extreme discomfort.

Dosage: One 5-grain aspirin tablet per 20 pounds body weight, to a maximum of 5 tablets (25 grains) per day. (See How to Administer Tablets and Pills.)

Anthropomorphism

Next to sheer ignorance, anthropomorphism is probably the second-ranking cause of improper home medical treatment. Anthropomorphism in this context is the fallacy of attributing human behavior and mentality to dogs.

While it is perfectly normal to speak of an animal as being "nearly human," actually believing it can lead to serious errors in judgment, which in turn can lead to incorrect medical treatment. If we think of a dog as a human being, we cannot properly observe and evaluate the animal's behavior. In many instances, this makes it impossible to reach a correct diagnosis.

Dogs have their own psychology, their own behavior patterns, and their own set of reactions. If we are to treat dogs intelligently, we must think of them as dogs, and not as four-legged people.

Antibiotics and Antibiotic Treatment

Antibiotics are drugs that kill or inhibit the growth of germs that cause certain infections. They are most effective when administered during the early growth stage of the infection. Antibiotics are usually ineffective against virus infections.

Ideally, if your dog develops an infectious disease, the particular strain of bacteria responsible should be identified and the specific antibiotic administered.

Unfortunately, disease states are rarely ideal, so a broad-spectrum antibiotic is administered while a specific germ is being identified.

If there is no response within twenty-four hours, another broad-spectrum antibiotic is used, and possibly another, until a satisfactory response occurs.

Artificial Respiration

Artificial respiration does the work of normal breathing: shifting air into and out of the dog's lungs. It should be administered as soon as one observes that the animal is not breathing. Delay can be fatal. Five minutes after breathing stops, the animal will be beyond recovery.

Technique: Lay the dog on its right side. Open the

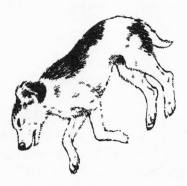

animal's mouth and check to be sure that there are no obstructions to breathing. If there are obstructions (e.g., sand, gravel, etc.), pull them out with your finger. Make sure that the tongue is lolling out, clear of the back of the

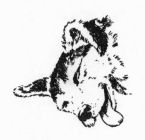

throat. Place the flat of both hands below the shoulder blade and over the ribs. Press down firmly to empty the

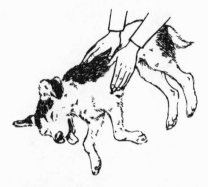

lungs. Release the pressure. The lungs should fill as the

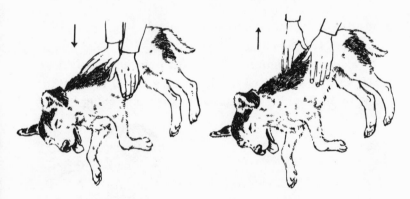

natural elasticity of the chest returns it to its normal position. Repeat pressing down and releasing the pressure every five seconds until the dog is breathing on its own again. This could take up to an hour. The movements should be brisk and forceful. Press down hard. Release suddenly.

Mouth-to-nostrils resuscitation: Hold the dog's mouth closed and blow into its nostrils. Wait a second and blow

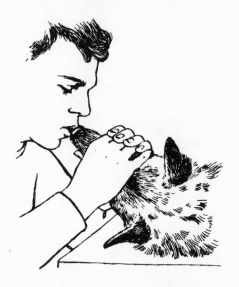

again. The idea is to inflate the animal's lungs with air so that they function of their own accord.

Swinging technique: Used with pups and small dogs. Slap the dog sharply on the side once or twice. Then lift the dog by its hind legs, extend your arms, and swing it back

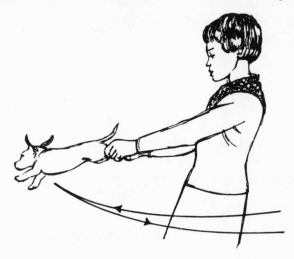

and forth ten times. Wait a few seconds for a gasp. If there is none, swing the animal again.

When you swing a dog in this way, the weight of the abdominal contents will contract and expand the lungs. If, after four such swinging sessions, the dog is still not breathing, administer mouth-to-mouth resuscitation.

Bandaging: General

Bandages are used to: stop bleeding, support injured legs; prevent the dog from biting at its injuries; reduce swelling; prevent bacteria from entering a wound and causing infection.

Preferred type of bandage: The easiest type of bandage to use is the Ace ® bandage, available in twelve- and fifteen-foot lengths and in a variety of widths. For bandaging dogs, the most useful is the two- or three-inch width. For wounds on the trunk of the dog, the five-inch bandage is suggested. It is sensible to keep a few different types of bandages in a handy first aid kit, but in emergencies any wad of material will do.

Bandaging the Ear

Ears are rather difficult to bandage, but unfortunately dog owners have ample opportunity to practice. A dog's ears are frequently torn after fights with other dogs and tend to bleed profusely, especially when the injured animal shakes its head.

Technique: Place a pad of absorbent cotton on top of the dog's head. Fold the affected ear over the pad. Place

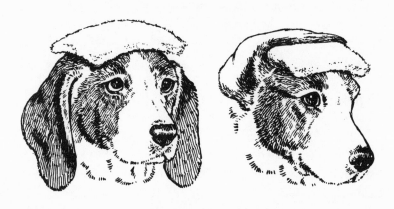

another pad of absorbent cotton over the ear. Wind the

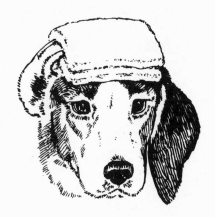

bandage around the head several times, leaving the unaffected ear in its normal position. Anchor the bandage with

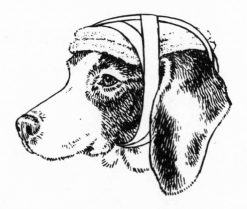

a strip of two- or three-inch adhesive tape placed on the top of the head. Care must be taken to ensure that the bandage

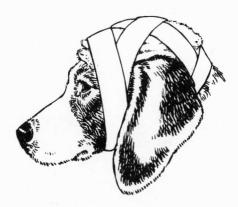

is not wound too tightly, and does not affect the animal's breathing.

Bandaging the Eye

Technique: Place a moist gauze pad over the affected eye. Wind the bandage around the dog's head, leaving the

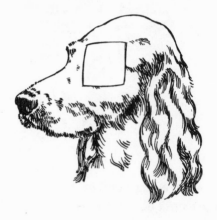

ears in their normal position. Extend the bandage forward

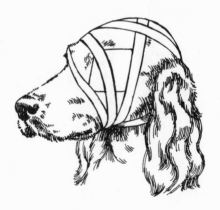

to cover the gauze dressing over the affected eye. Anchor

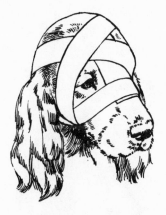

the bandage with a strip of two- or three-inch adhesive tape, placed at the top of the dog's head. Take care not to

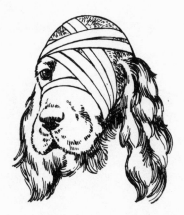

wind the bandage too tightly, and be sure that it does not interfere with the dog's breathing.

Bandaging the Leg

Technique: When bandaging the leg, bandage the foot as well, to prevent swelling and tissue damage. Pack the spaces between the dog's toes with small wads of absorbent cotton to prevent damage to the toes. Wrap absorbent

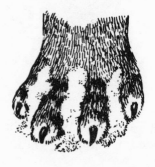

cotton around the foot. Begin bandaging at the top of the

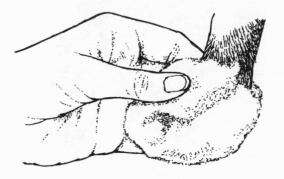

leg, go down the front of the leg, around the foot, and up

the back. Then wind the bandage around the leg, each layer

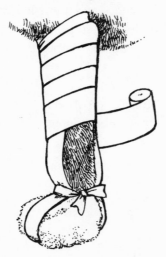

of bandage overlapping the preceding layer, until the whole leg is covered. Tie off the bandage.

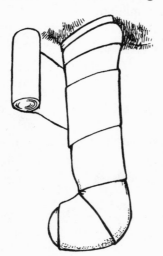

The bandage should be wound firmly enough not to slip, but not so tightly that it stops the circulation, unless it is a pressure bandage intended to stop a hemorrhage. In that case, it should be loosened and tightened again every thirty minutes until the bleeding stops. Do not unwind the bandage completely, or you may reopen the wound.

Body Weight—(Knowledge of body weight is often necessary for determining correct dosage of medicines.)

Hounds

Afghan hound	60+ lbs.
Basenji	21-25 lbs.
Basset hound	40-50 lbs.
Beagle	20-40 lbs.
Bloodhound	80-90 lbs.
Borzoi	60+ lbs.
Dachshund (standard)	25 lbs.
Dachshund (miniature)	11 lbs.
Deerhound	85-105 lbs.
Norwegian elkhound	50 lbs.
Finnish spitz	40 lbs.
Foxhound	70 lbs.
Greyhound	60-70 lbs.
Harrier	70 lbs.
Irish wolfhound	120+ lbs.
Otterhound	65 lbs.
Rhodesian ridgeback	85 lbs.
Saluki	50 lbs.
Whippet	20 lbs.

Terriers

Airedale terrier	50+ lbs.
Australian terrier	10+ lbs.

Bedlington terrier	18-23 lbs.
Border terrier	13-15½ lbs.
Bull terrier (miniature)	20 lbs.
Cairn terrier	14 lbs.
Dandie Dinmont terrier	18 lbs.
Fox terrier (smooth)	16-18 lbs.
Fox terrier (wire-haired)	16-18 lbs.
Irish terrier	27 lbs.
Kerry blue terrier	30-40 lbs.
Lakeland terrier	17 lbs.
Manchester terrier	20 lbs.
Norfolk terrier	15 lbs.
Norwich terrier	12 lbs.
Scottish terrier	19-23 lbs.
Sealyham terrier	18-20 lbs.
Skye terrier	24-30 lbs.
Staffordshire bull terrier	28-38 lbs.
Welsh terrier	20 lbs.
West Highland white terrier	15-18 lbs.

Toy Dogs

Chihuahua (long-haired)	6 lbs.
Chihuahua (smooth coat)	6 lbs.
English toy terrier	8 lbs.
Belgian griffon	6-9 lbs.
Italian greyhound	6-8 lbs.
Japanese	4-9 lbs.
King Charles spaniel	10-18 lbs.
Maltese	5-7 lbs.
Miniature pinscher	10 lbs.
Papillon	3-7 lbs.
Pekingese	7-12 lbs.
Pomeranian	3-5 lbs.

Poodle	up to 10 lbs.
Pug	14-18 lbs.
Yorkshire terrier	up to 7 lbs.

Gundogs

English setter	60 lbs.
Gordon setter	65 lbs.
Irish setter (red)	60 lbs.
Pointer	50-55 lbs.
German short-haired pointer	45-70 lbs.
Labrador retriever	70 lbs.
Clumber spaniel	55-70 lbs.
Cocker spaniel	25-28 lbs.
Field spaniel	35 lbs.
Irish water slaniel	30-40 lbs.
English springer spaniel	40-50 lbs.
Sussex spaniel	45 lbs.
Weimaraner	45-65 lbs.

Nonsporting Dogs

Alsatian (German shepherd)	up to 90 lbs.
Bearded collie	up to 50 lbs.
Boston terrier	15-25 lbs.
Boxer	60 lbs.
Bulldog	50-55 lbs.
Bull mastiff	110-130 lbs.
Chow chow	60 lbs.
Collie (rough)	50 lbs.
Collie (smooth)	50 lbs.
Dalmatian	50-55 lbs.
Doberman pinscher	60-100 lbs.
French bulldog	28 lbs.
Great Dane	120+ lbs.
Keeshond	40 lbs.

Lhasa apso	12-15 lbs.
Mastiff	120+ lbs.
Newfoundland	150 lbs.
Poodle (standard)	50+ lbs.
Poodle (miniature)	10 lbs.
Great Pyrenees	100-125 lbs.
St. Bernard	120+ lbs.
Samoyed	45-55 lbs.
Shipperke	12-16 lbs.
Schnauzer (standard)	30 lbs.
Schnauzer (miniature)	15 lbs.
Old English sheepdog	80-100 lbs.
Shetland sheepdog	10 lbs.
Shih Tzu	14-16 lbs.
Tibetan spaniel	9-16 lbs.
Tibetan terrier	14-30 lbs.
Welsh corgi (Pembroke)	20-24 lbs.
Welsh corgi (Cardigan)	22-26 lbs.

Car Accidents

First consideration: Do not move the animal any more than you have to. Decide where you are going to move the dog before you move it.

Moving an injured dog: Small dogs may be lifted by the scruff of the neck and carried. The best way to move a large dog is on an improvised stretcher. The backseat of a car will serve. If there is no one to help you carry the stretcher, make a sling using your coat or a blanket and carry the animal in it.

Moving an animal in great pain is not the easiest thing to do, so be prepared for some problems. A badly hurt or frightened dog may bite anyone who tries to touch it, including its owner. Do not waste time trying to calm the dog with soothing talk: if it is really hurt, it will not hear you. Just take the proper precautions against being bitten and get on with the job.

Technique for tying tape muzzle: The best way to prevent a dog from biting you while giving it treatment is to tie its jaws shut. If the animal is hysterical, that is what you will have to do. Use a short length of cord, a necktie or, if there is one, a bandage. Loop this around the muzzle and make the first knot anywhere well back on the dog's mouth, out of biting range. Then cross the remaining lengths around the muzzle again and make another knot, this one under the jaw. Carry the bandage back behind the dog's neck and tie the final knot just behind its ears. Now you can safely handle the dog. (See Restraint and Handling.)

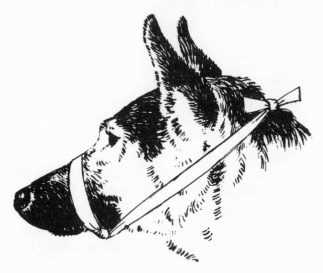

Slide, do not lift, the animal onto the stretcher or into the sling and get it to the nearest vet. It is much better and faster to get the dog to the vet than to try to get the vet to the dog. If possible, have someone telephone the vet so that emergency treatment is ready when you arrive.

If you do not know a vet, call the police; they will tell you where the dog should be taken.

Warmth, no fluids: Try to keep the dog warm while you are getting it to the vet. Do not apply external heat. To prevent loss of body heat, keep the animal covered with a coat or a blanket. Do not try to numb the pain by pouring whiskey down the dog's throat. Do not try to counteract shock with warm milk or water.

Bleeding: If the dog is bleeding badly, try to stop or at least stanch the bleeding. If you can, determine whether the animal is bleeding from an artery or a vein. This is done by observing the way the blood flows.

Arterial wounds: If the blood comes out in a pumping fashion, in time with the heartbeat, and if it is bright red, then it is from an artery. The bleeding must be stopped immediately or the dog will die.

For arteries, if the wound is on the limbs, make a tourniquet by wrapping a bandage, handkerchief, or necktie around the limb, *above* the injury, and inserting a pencil or screwdriver into the bandage, on the side of the wound nearest the heart. Then twist the tourniquet until the bleeding stops. (See Tourniquets.)

Venous wounds: Blood flowing from a vein flows regularly, as opposed to being pumped from an artery. It is dark red. If the blood is coming from a vein, apply the tourniquet *below* the wound.

It's important to remember that a tourniquet be just tight enough to stop the bleeding. Loosen the tourniquet every ten minutes to allow the blood to get to the rest of the leg.

Bleeding emergencies: Unfortunately, is is usually such a gory mess that you cannot always determine whether the blood is flowing or pumping. Often the wounds are on a part of the body where a tourniquet cannot be applied. So, unless the source of blood is obvious and can be easily tied off, the best thing you can do is the fastest thing you can do. Grab anything—bandages, a torn shirt, a handkerchief, even a package of tissues—and put it over the wound, holding it there with as much pressure as you can.

Internal bleeding: If the bleeding is internal, or the blood is flowing from the dog's nose or anus, keep the animal still and get it to a vet as fast as possible. (Try not to have another accident while you are rushing the dog to the vet.)

Further attempts at first aid will almost certainly do more harm than good. Broken or fractured bones need expert treatment. Leave that treatment to an expert. Concentrate on getting the injured dog to the expert.

Clipping Nails

Buy nail clippers at a pet store. If the nail is black and

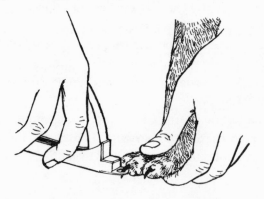

the quick cannot be seen, cut along the line formed by the base of the nail.

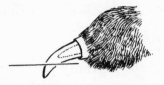

Warning: Do not clip the nail too short or you will cut the vein under the nail and cause the toe to bleed.

Should this happen, the bleeding can be controlled by bandaging the nail (see Bandaging: General), or by applying a silver nitrate pencil (from drugstore) to the site of the bleeding. (Wear rubber gloves when you are using the silver nitrate pencil to avoid burning your fingers.)

Compresses—Hot and Cold

A compress is made by taking a wad of absorbent cotton or material and saturating it in the proper solution.

Cold compresses or ice packs are applied directly over a swelling caused by a blow, and will reduce the swelling.

Hot compresses are especially effective for relieving pain. They are made by soaking the cotton in the hottest water your hands can bear. Wring out the excess water and apply to the affected area for about two minutes. Repeat as often as possible.

Hot compresses relieve pain.

Cold compresses reduce swelling.

Hot and cold compresses can be used in conjunction with each other. For sprains and strains, alternate hot and cold compresses.

Cough Medicines

A cough medicine is a product designed to soothe or suppress a cough.

Before administering cough medicines, bear in mind that a cough is not a separate entity, but a possible symptom of many diseases.

A cough medicine may stop the cough temporarily and allow the dog to rest, but it will not cure whatever is causing the cough. If possible, try to determine the cause of the cough before administering the medicine.

Possible causes of coughs: Tonsillitis; laryngitis; bronchitis; pneumonia; pleurisy; foreign body in throat; distemper; chronic heart disease; heartworm infestation.

Treatment: A homemade solution of 2 tablespoons honey and 1 teaspoon lemon juice in 2 tablespoons water, or any human cough syrup: one to two teaspoons per 20 pounds body weight three times a day.

If the dog is still coughing after 24 hours, consult a vet.

Destruction

Animals in their natural wild state rarely die of old age. Having extended the life span of our dogs by protecting them insofar as possible from illness and accident, we have the responsibility of caring for them in their old age and, finally, of sparing them any unnecessary suffering.

A part of that responsibility is deciding when that point of unnecessary suffering has been reached. Chronic illness, incontinence, and senility are factors to be balanced against more subjective feelings such as the dog owner's love for his pet and the sanctity of life in general.

Although the final decision is the individual dog owner's responsibility, all too often people permit their pets to linger on painfully, hoping that the poor old thing will die soon. When you find yourself feeling that way, perhaps it is time to do your dog one last kindness.

When a dog is put to sleep by a veterinarian, the process is simple and painless. The dog is given an injection of an anesthetic. Before you can count to three, the dog is dead. Its troubles, aches, and pains are over.

The most difficult situations arise when a dog has been badly injured—usually in an auto accident—and is in great pain. Most people are not equipped, mentally or physically, to destroy the animal. So, rather than take the chance of causing even greater pain, call the police at once. They will give you the emergency phone number of the nearest vet. Leave this sad job to him.

Diet

An adequate diet is one that, when fed regularly, will maintain good health without the development of deficiency diseases and is palatable. However, dog owners tend to feed their dogs foods which are convenient to stock and easy to prepare, without regard to nutritional requirements. Dogs are accommodating animals: they will eat what you give them and will maintain a reasonable nutritional level for the most part.

This does not mean that a dog can be fed anything. Convenience is fine, but a well-balanced diet is essential. A well-balanced diet should contain the correct proportions of: proteins; carbohydrates; fats; minerals; and vitamins. (See Nutrition.) Dogs can be fed either commercial preparations or fresh foods prepared by the owner. Proprietary foods are either canned or dried meats, biscuits or kibbles, or semi-dry cakes. Home-prepared foods are usually raw or cooked meats and some biscuit meal.

For orphan puppies, pregnant bitches, lactating bitches, sick dogs, old dogs, and nephritic dogs, see the appropriate sections.

Docking and Cropping

Cropping refers to cutting and reshaping dogs' ears. Docking means shortening, again by cutting, dogs' tails.

The cropping of dogs' ears is illegal in Britain, but in other parts of Europe and in the United States the docking and cropping of certain breeds is customary.

In the authors' opinion, these procedures are nothing more than mutilation dictated by fashion. Further, docking a tail may cause chronic problems in the anal area. However, if the owner insists upon docking or cropping, the operation should be performed by a qualified person.

Elizabethan Collar

A most useful device when treating cuts, skin diseases, etc., an Elizabethan collar is used to prevent a dog from scratching at its face, ears, or eyes, or to prevent it from biting various parts of its anatomy.

Classically, these collars are prepared from stiff cardboard; but this has obvious disadvantages, and we recommend plastic containers varying in size from a small flowerpot for a small pup to a large plastic basket for a large dog.

Cut the bottom out of the flowerpot to a size that the head will go through. Punch four more holes around this hole, put strings through, and tie the "collar" to the dog's collar.

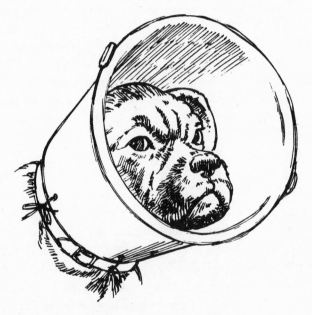

The open end must be far enough away from the nose to prevent licking, and this may present difficulties at feeding time. If so, the collar can be removed briefly to allow eating and drinking. The Elizabethan collar may sound and even look a bit uncomfortable, but most dogs accept them quite calmly after the first few minutes.

Emetics (Induced Vomiting)

An emetic is any substance that induces vomiting, and it is usually given after a dog has eaten something poisonous. (See Poisoning: General.)

Table salt: Table salt is a suitable emetic for dogs. It is a good idea to keep a small container in your first aid kit. Take 1 tablespoon of the dry salt crystals and throw them as far back down the animal's throat as you can see. (See How to Administer Tablets and Pills.)

To be effective, the emetic must be administered as soon as possible after the dog has eaten the poison. If the poison has been consumed more than an hour previously, or if the dog is shocked or drowsy, do not induce vomiting.

Warning: Never attempt to make an unconscious animal vomit.

Enemas

An enema is an injection of nonirritant fluid into the large intestine, administered by way of the anal passage. The purpose of giving an enema is to empty the large intestine of any abnormal or impacted contents, so that the dog can have a normal bowel movement. Enemas may be necessary after the consumption of a large amount of bones (not recommended feeding).

How to prepare an enema: The best enema solution is produced by lathering some good quality soap into a dishpan of warm water (1 pint warm water with soap or soap flakes that contain no detergent). This solution is administered into the anal passage by means of an enema bag.

If an enema bag is not available you can improvise, using a length of rubber tubing (approximately ⅓ inch in diameter) leading to a plastic funnel or container (e.g., a plastic dish with a hole punched in it) filled with the enema solution.

Technique: Spread some newspapers around the area *before* you give the enema; you will not have time afterwards. Have someone hold the dog. (See Restraint.) Enemas should only be given with the dog standing. Introduce about three inches of tubing into the dog's rectum. A little Vaseline ® on the end of the tubing helps. Hold the container higher than the dog.

Dosage: Administer 2–3 fluid ounces for a small dog, up to 1 pint for a large dog.

If the substances causing impaction are not passed after three attempts, professional help should be sought.

Feeding Times

Dogs should be fed regularly at the same hour each day. In this respect they are creatures of habit, and at the accustomed hour their gastric juices begin to flow.

Puppies: Puppies should receive several meals a day: at eight weeks, feed four times a day; fourteen weeks, three times a day; eighteen weeks, two times a day; six months, one meal a day.

Adult dogs: Grown dogs may be fed once or twice a day, depending upon the dog's appetite and the amount of exercise. Elderly dogs should be fed two or even three smaller meals, rather than one large one.

First Aid Kit

All dog owners should prepare a first aid kit and keep it in a clearly marked container in a safe place. It should contain:

A pair of sharp-edged, blunt-pointed scissors.
A pair of forceps (tweezers).
Four rolls of two-inch adhesive tape.
Four rolls of two-inch Ace ® roller bandage.
A package of absorbent cotton.
A package of gauze.
A bottle of antiseptic (e.g., pHisoDerm ®, iodine).
A razor blade.
An eyedropper.
A package of needles.
Aspirin tablets.
Acetaminophen.
A package of cotton buds.
Milk of magnesia.
Table salt.
A copy of this book.
The vet's address and phone number.

Force-Feeding

To force-feed solid food, break the food into small pellets and feed them exactly as you would administer a tablet or pill; that is, hold the dog's muzzle with your left hand, thumb on one side, the rest of your fingers on the other side. With the index finger of your right hand, press down on the lower incisors; then place the pellet far back in the dog's mouth and hold its mouth shut. Stroke its throat until it swallows. Then begin again.

When force-feeding a fluid, pull the pouch formed at the side of the dog's lip out a little with your finger and pour the fluid, a bit at a time, into the pouch. Close the pouch, and hold it closed while you stroke the animal's throat until it swallows. Repeat.

Glucose (Dextrose monohydrate)

This is a type of sugar which serves as a source of quick energy, to be given when the dog is weak and apathetic. Sprinkle the powder on the food or put it into the water.

Substitute: If a glucose powder is not available, a substitute mixture can be made by adding 2 tablespoons sugar to 1 pint water and stirring until the sugar has dissolved.

Grooming

Most dogs groom themselves, but the wise dog owner does not leave the job entirely to the animal. The act of grooming not only helps the dog keep clean, but it establishes a physical rapport between dog and owner. This rapport will stand the owner in good stead on those occasions when it is necessary to handle the dog in order to administer medical treatment.

Healthy dogs will do their best to keep their coats clean, but even the most zealous dog is unable to keep up with the city's accumulation of grime. It is well to remember that our dogs live in a world six inches to three feet in height, about level with a car exhaust pipe.

City dogs should be bathed once a month. Small dogs can be put in a tub; larger dogs, with an aversion to baths, should be washed with a hose. If it is a large dog living in a small apartment, where hosing is not practical, then the tub will have to be used. An assistant is helpful in this case. Also, be prepared to get wet. Even though many dogs, like small children, dislike baths, they can be bathed against their wishes. Be determined, be firm. Know what you are going to do, and get on with it. (See How to Shampoo a Dog).

How to Administer Tablets and Pills

Concealment: If the dog is not being starved, conceal the pill or tablet in a tasty tidbit such as meat or cheese. However, some dogs are notorious for finding even the most cunningly concealed pill. In this case, be prepared to administer the pill directly.

Direct technique: Place your left hand on top of the dog's head, with your thumb and index finger placed behind the canine teeth. Pull the dog's head upward. The tablet is

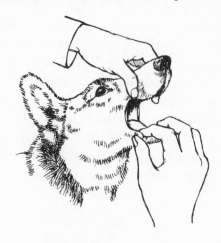

in your right hand. Use this hand to open the dog's mouth by holding the lower jaw behind the lower canine teeth.

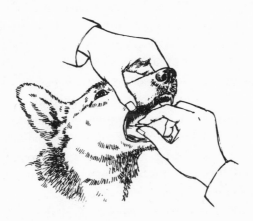

Push the tablet as far down the dog's throat as possible. Hold the dog's jaw shut until it swallows.

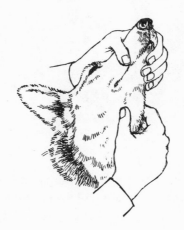

How to Give an Injection

While it is not usual for dog owners to administer injections, there are occasional situations, such as diabetes or certain long courses of antibiotic treatment, when knowledge of the technique can be very useful.

The subcutaneous injection is an injection under the skin, as opposed to the intravenous injection, which is directly into the vein. The subcutaneous injection is relatively simple to administer and completely painless.

When administering an injection, be confident and self-assured. If you are hesitant, the dog will sense it and the process will be that much more difficult.

Technique: If there is someone available, ask him to hold your dog for you. If there is a possibility that the dog might bite, tape its muzzle. Saturate a pad of absorbent

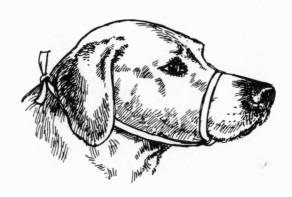

cotton with alcohol and swab the skin around the scruff of the neck, where the injection will be administered. Do not make a great show of this, or you will alarm the dog.

A quick rub with the cotton is sufficient. After filling the syringe, hold it point uppermost and slowly press the plunger until all the air is out of the syringe. Hold the

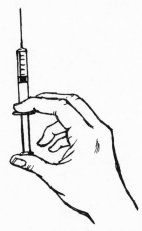

syringe at the base, between your index finger and thumb. With your other hand, lift a fold of skin at the scruff of the neck into a cone, and slip the needle under the skin below the cone. Press the plunger. Keep the needle as nearly parallel with the skin surface as possible. When the con-

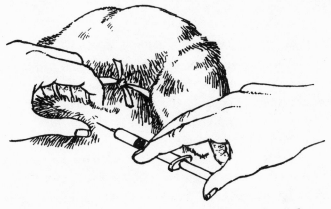

tents of the syringe have been injected, withdraw the syringe and rub the site of the injection for a few seconds to make certain that the fluid has been dispersed.

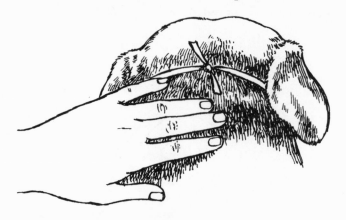

If an assistant is not available, you can easily hold most animals by the scruff of the neck with one hand while administering the injection with the other. By holding the animal by the scruff of the neck, you also minimize the danger of being bitten.

How to Open a Dog's Mouth

There are two ways of opening a dog's mouth:

(1) With your left hand placed far back on the dog's muzzle, thumb on one side of the muzzle, other fingers on the other side, you hold the dog's head. Then place the index finger of your right hand on the lower incisor teeth and pry open the dog's mouth.

(2) With smaller dogs, the one-handed method is simply to grip the muzzle as far back as you can, and with your thumb on one side and the other fingers on the other side, press firmly on the hinge of the jaws.

How to Shampoo a Dog

Wet the dog thoroughly. Lather a good-quality hand soap or mild shampoo into the dog's coat. Wash all the lather out of the dog's coat. Be careful not to get any soap in the dog's eyes, or you will find it twice as difficult the next time you try to give the animal a bath.

Contrary to a widely held belief, frequent washing does not remove the oils from the coat; rather it stimulates production of these natural oils. If skin conditions are present, use a selenium disulfide shampoo.

In addition to monthly baths, dogs should be given a good brushing every day. The long-haired breeds should be combed as well as brushed to prevent tangling. Any knots of tangled hair that do not comb out should be cut out with scissors.

Warning: If the dog's grooming is neglected, and its coat is allowed to become filthy and matted, the dog will develop a predisposition for skin diseases.

Grooming sick animals: The importance of grooming as a factor in nursing, contributing to the dog's well-being, cannot be overemphasized. Sick dogs may neglect their grooming. They have an excuse; their owners do not. Apart from the coat, keep the eyes, nose, ears, and area around the mouth clean by wiping regularly with a little diluted pHisoHex ® on absorbent cotton (1 teaspoon pHisoHex to 10 teaspoons water). A dog with diarrhea will develop a sore anus. Treat this soreness by applying cold cream or baby diaper rash cream.

If it is not desirable to bathe a dog in water, there are several "dry bath" preparations available. These are in the form of powder which is dusted into the dog's coat and then brushed out. Although dry shampoos are convenient, they are not as effective as wet shampoos.

Longevity

Perhaps the saddest thing about owning and loving a dog is the brevity of a dog's life span compared to our own.

Large breeds: The larger breeds generally have the shortest life span; seven or eight years is a ripe old age for a Great Dane.

Small breeds: Smaller dogs are often still fit at the age of thirteen or fourteen years.

Nursing: General Care of Sick Dogs

If your dog is suffering from a severe or debilitating disease and is too weak and too sick to groom and feed itself, the nursing and loving care it receives from you will have a vital effect upon recovery.

This nursing care extends to grooming and hygiene as well as to proper feeding. Keep sick dogs in a warm, quiet, dimly lit place. Try not to disturb them. Keep sick dogs clean. Special care should be taken if they are suffering from diarrhea or vomiting, for psychological as well as sanitary reasons. All animals are fastidious and become distressed if allowed to foul themselves. If this occurs, they should be gently washed with soap and water. A dusting of talcum powder after washing is helpful. Larger dogs, if too weak to move themselves, should be turned regularly, every four hours, to avoid bedsores.

Apart from your doing what is necessary for their

well-being, sick dogs should be left alone as much as possible. There is a difference between loving care and fussing. Do not fuss over a sick dog.

Diet: Sick dogs and dogs recuperating from an illness need nourishing food even if they don't always want it. Supplement their diet with a mixture of 4 tablespoons glucose to 1 pint water, daily, to supply extra energy. Do not give this, or any fluids, to a dog that is vomiting. (See Excessive Thirst.)

If the dog has an appetite, do not give the animal all that it wants at one time. Feed it smaller amounts at frequent intervals.

If the dog has no appetite, try to tempt it with strong-smelling foods such as cheese or canned sardines. A dog's sense of smell, if properly enticed, will often start it eating again. Homemade meat extracts often do the trick. These extracts are made by mincing raw meat as finely as possible and pouring boiling water over it. The resulting liquid is then poured into a bowl, with a pinch of salt and a pinch of monosodium glutamate added to bring out the flavor.

Make every effort to tempt the dog to eat voluntarily. If nothing works, you will have to force-feed. This is a last resort. Remember, the smallest amount of food taken voluntarily will do more good than a much larger amount that has been forced down. (See Force-Feeding.)

Hygiene: All bowls, dishes, spoons, etc., that come in contact with the dog must be sterilized in boiling water after each meal. Scrupulous hygiene is absolutely essential to successful nursing.

Nursing Diabetic Dogs (See Diabetes Mellitus)

The diabetic dog requires a diet that is high in protein and low in carbohydrates. Fortunately, most canned animal foods are of this composition and provide adequate nourishment when supplemented with two raw eggs per week. Mix the raw eggs into the dog's food to provide the necessary amount of fat. Do not give biscuits or cereal.

Nursing Elderly Dogs

Elderly dogs present special problems and their general condition can be greatly improved by feeding them good quality food in proper amounts. (See Excessive Appetite; Weight Gain; Diet.)

When nursing an older dog whose appetite is sluggish, stimulate the appetite by feeding meat extracts and flavorings. Since a dog's sense of smell and taste diminish with age, extra attention to diet is necessary to keep the sick elderly animal eating.

Most elderly dogs are nephritic, that is, they suffer from kidney problems, and should be fed an easily assimilated diet of white meat (fish or chicken) with carbohydrates, in the form of rice or dog biscuits, mixed into their food. Supplement the older dog's diet with Vitamin A capsules and vitamin B_{12} tablets (available at drugstores).

Elderly dogs should be given all the water they require; be sure the dog's drinking dish is always full.

Nursing Young Dogs: Birth to Six Months

Diet is of paramount importance in the successful nursing of young dogs. When dogs develop infections, their food intake falls. This is particularly dangerous with pups, which are very dependent upon daily nutrition. When they stop eating, they set in motion a cycle of malnutrition and further infection that ultimately ends in death.

A young dog weighing two pounds requires at least 8 teaspoons of water daily. In addition, it needs a diet containing minerals, protein, carbohydrates, fats, and vitamins. (See Diet.)

As long as there is *no diarrhea or vomiting,* add powdered cow's milk, at twice the strength recommended for human babies, to the puppy's diet.

For orphan puppies, milk substitutes may be given. Feed every two hours for the first week, day and night; afterwards, every three hours for ten days.

If there is diarrhea or vomiting, neither milk nor milk products should be given. Withhold all food for twelve hours, then make a mixture of 1 cup water, 3 tablespoons glucose, 1 raw egg white, 1 pinch salt. Give 2 tablespoons every two hours. Small portions of deboned chicken or fish may be given three or four times a day for four days.

If the puppy still refuses to eat after twenty-four hours, contact a vet.

Nutrition

To maintain good health, dogs require a diet that includes carbohydrates, fats, proteins, minerals, and vitamins in the proper proportions. The simplest adequate ration is raw meat containing about 10% fat, plus an equal amount of cereal in the form of dog biscuits. Cooked, deboned fish can be substituted for meat. Cornmeal or oatmeal can be used as an alternative to dog biscuits.

Canned foods mixed with an equal amount of cereal may be used in place of raw meat. These canned foods are more expensive but more convenient. If canned foods are used, supplement them occasionally with a piece of fresh meat, particularly liver, to ensure proper vitamin intake.

An adequate canned dog food will contain: 13% protein; 5% fat; 16% carbohydrate; 2.5% ash.

Feeding amounts:

Size of dog	Body weight	Food intake
Small	10 pounds	up to ½ pound
Medium	25 pounds	1¼ pounds
Large	40 pounds	1¾ pounds
Very large	100 pounds	2½ pounds and over

This guide to feeding amounts is based on a mixed diet made up of 50% meat or meat substitutes and 50% meal or cereal. Further, this guide assumes that the dog is getting enough exercise. If this is not the case, the food supply should be reduced proportionately, up to half the normal amount for sedentary or elderly dogs. (See also Diet.)

Orphan Puppies

Very young puppies (up to four weeks old) without a mother, or those from a mother unable to breast-feed them (see Agalactia), should be placed in a small, warm box and fed a substitute milk supplement every two hours for the first two weeks (day and night). After that, feed every three hours.

After each feeding, burp the puppies by rubbing their abdomens gently with an oiled finger. This burping is normally accompanied by urination and defecation.

Homemade milk supplement: If commercial substitutes are not available, you can make your own milk supplement by combining: 30 ounces cow's milk, 1 egg yolk, 1 pinch bone meal, 1 pinch citric acid. Stir the mixture and keep it in the refrigerator. Warm it to 100°F. before feeding.

Feeding technique: Use an eyedropper or doll's feeding bottle. Be sure to thoroughly clean and then boil the dropper or doll's bottle after each feeding. The amount of food required will vary with the size of the puppies. Generally, they should be fed according to their appetites. Unfortunately, some puppies have appetites larger than their capacity.

Diarrhea: Overfeeding may result in *diarrhea*. Should diarrhea develop, withhold all milk supplement and give the puppy lukewarm boiled water with glucose added—3 tablespoons glucose to 1 pint boiled water—for two feedings. If the diarrhea stops, return to the milk supplement. If the diarrhea persists for more than twenty-four hours, call a vet. If the diarrhea was not caused by overfeeding, it may be the result of an infection.

Solid foods: After three weeks, pups will show an interest in more adult food. Encourage this new appetite by feeding them bits of deboned chicken, fish, and chopped meat.

Weaning: Taking the young puppies off their mother's milk or off the milk supplement should be completed by the time the puppies are four to five weeks old.

Poultices

Use: The prolonged application of heat to a swelling or to a sore area will relieve the pain and control the swelling. The advantage of a poultice is that it retains heat without having to be changed constantly. There are several types of poultices but the simplest and one of the most effective is the kaolin poultice.

Prepare the poultice by heating the can of kaolin (available at drugstores) in a saucepan of boiling water. When the clay is fairly hot, spread it on a bandage and tape the bandage over the affected area. Before placing the bandage on the dog, test a bit of the kaolin on the back of your hand. It should be very warm, but not hot enough to cause any pain. The poultice should be changed every four hours.

Substitutes: If kaolin is not available, a poultice may be made from bread or potatoes. To make a poultice from bread: boil some water, soak a piece of bread in the boiling water, allow it to cool enough for you to handle it, then apply it to the affected area. To make a poultice from potatoes: mash some cooked potatoes and apply them to the affected area.

Pulse Rate and Average Rectal Temperature

Normal pulse rate for dogs: 80–120 beats a minute. As a general rule, the smaller the breed or species, the higher the pulse rate.

Average rectal temperature for dogs: 101.3°F.

Restraint and Handling

By restraint we mean the technique of handling, moving, and holding a dog, usually against its will.

When to use restraint: When one must do something which the dog finds frightening, painful, or objectionable. It is never pleasant to use restraint, but when it is necessary, be firm, unhurried, and know what you are going to do before you approach the dog.

There are several methods of restraining reluctant dogs. The method you use depends upon: the size of the dog, and your purpose in restraining the dog. Do you want to move the animal or hold it?

Techniques: The first step in restraining a dog is to make sure that it does not bite you. The easiest way to do this is to tie its mouth closed. Take a bandage or necktie, wrap it around the dog's nose several times, then tie the free ends around its neck behind the ears.

The dog may then be held by your putting an arm around its neck. With your other arm, grasp the dog around

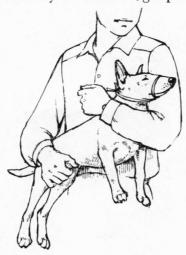

the hips. Hold the animal against your body to prevent it from wriggling out of your arms.

Small dogs: Small dogs or those with short noses are more difficult to restrain, but they can be handled by having a rolled towel wrapped around their necks. A variation of

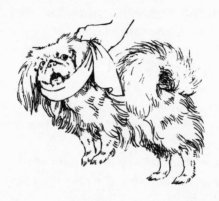

this technique is to get behind the dog, grab the scruff of its neck with one hand, grab its back legs with your other hand and stretch them.

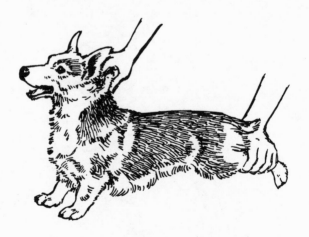

Large dogs: Get behind the dog, grab it firmly by the skin of the neck, just behind the head, with one hand on one side of the head and the other hand on the other side. Now the dog may be either held or dragged.

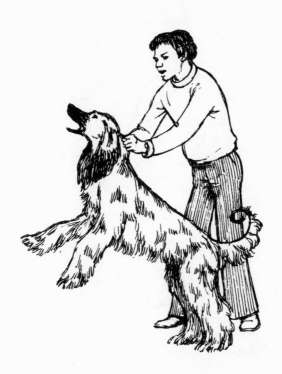

Saline Solution

A sterile (germ-free) salt solution, used to wash eyes, wounds, etc.

Dissolve 1 teaspoon iodine-free table salt in 1 pint boiling water. Allow the water to cool to body temperature, then apply.

Taking the Pulse

Technique: Place your index and middle fingers over the femoral artery at the point where it crosses the thigh bone on the inside of the thigh, almost in the groin. Count the

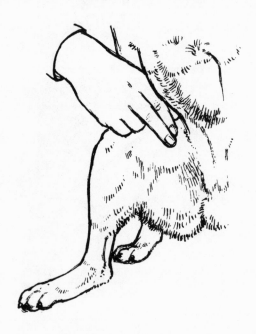

pulse beats for one minute. The smaller the dog, the faster the pulse rate, which, depending upon size and individual animal, varies from 80–120 beats a minute when the dog is in good health. In a dog running a high fever, the pulse rate may be as fast as 160 beats a minute. The dog owner should know his pet's normal pulse rate when the dog is in good health, so that a higher or lower rate will not go unnoticed.

Taking Samples of Feces and Urine

Technique: To assist your vet in diagnosing certain illnesses, a specimen of the dog's feces or urine will be needed. Since dogs do not always "perform" at the most convenient time and place, this may require some persistence on the owner's part.

The best time to collect the sample is first thing in the morning. Collect the sample of feces immediately and put it in a tin or can, clearly labeled with the dog's name, the owner's name and address, and the date.

Collecting a sample of urine requires even more persistence, especially with bitches! Do not try to collect the sample directly from the dog into a bottle. Use a sheet of plastic, shaped with a dent in the center. Let the dog smell the plastic before it urinates, so that it will not be too alarmed when you try to catch the urine in it. (A saucer or scallop shell may also be used, but you will have to be very quick.) As soon as the dog begins to pass water, place the plastic sheet in the best position to catch the urine, and then transfer it to a bottle. Make sure the bottle is clearly labeled. Fortunately, one does not need a great deal of urine for laboratory analysis. A few drops will be sufficient.

Taking Temperature

Most infectious and contagious diseases in the early stages cause the body temperature to rise. This rise is often, but not always, accompanied by lethargy and loss of appetite. Identification of fever and its severity provides the dog owner with a guide as to whether a vet should be consulted.

Taking a dog's temperature is not at all difficult. The technique is simple.

Type of thermometer: Any stubby, bulbed clinical thermometer may be used.

Technique: A dog's temperature must always be taken rectally. (If you put a thermometer in a dog's mouth, the animal will probably try to eat it.)

Have someone hold the dog while you take its temperature. If there is a possibility that the dog might bite, tie its muzzle (see Restraint and Handling), but a well-trained pet should allow its owner to take its temperature without making too much of a fuss.

Hold the thermometer by the end opposite the bulb, between your thumb and index finger, and then shake it with a sharp, jerky movement until the mercury is down to 95°F. On your first attempt, it is best to do it over a thick rug or bed, so that if you do drop the thermometer it will not break. Dip the bulb of the thermometer in Vaseline ®, cold cream, or baby oil. Approach the dog from the rear and gently slide an inch of the thermometer through the anal sphincter, using a gentle rotary action. Be prepared to stop the dog from trying to sit down. Push the thermometer in with a light touch, letting it find its own direction. When the thermometer is in place, support the protruding end very lightly and wait one full minute. Then withdraw the thermometer, wipe it clean with cotton or tissue, and read the temperature.

Reading a thermometer: All clinical thermometers are marked in degrees, with large marks and small marks for each one-fifth degree. After withdrawing the thermometer from your dog, hold it up to the light and, still holding it by the end opposite the bulb, roll it between your fingers until you see the silver band of mercury. Calculate the degree of temperature.

Normal body temperature: 101.3°F. A temperature of 102.5°F. and higher is significant and good reason to consult a vet. When calculating temperatures, remember that an excited or frightened dog has a higher body temperature than a relaxed one; so subtract one degree if this is the case. When you have finished using the thermometer, wash it in cold water. If you use the same thermometer on more than one animal, dip it into alcohol to prevent the transferring of bacteria.

Should the thermometer break while in the dog, take the dog to a vet. If a vet is not available, administer mineral oil: 1 tablespoon mineral oil orally, three times a day, until the thermometer is expelled with feces.

Tourniquets

The purpose of a tourniquet is to stop the flow of blood from a severed artery or vein.

In an emergency, a tourniquet can be improvised from many things: a necktie, belt, strip of material, shoelace; even a strip of plaited grass will serve.

If the dog is bleeding badly, try to stanch the bleeding so that you can observe the way the blood is flowing: this indicates whether the dog is bleeding from an artery or a vein.

Arterial wounds: If bright red blood comes out in a pumping fashion in time with the heartbeat, then it is an artery and the bleeding must be stopped quickly or the dog will die.

Treatment: For arterial wounds (on the limbs), make a

tourniquet by wrapping a bandage or belt around the limb, *above* the injury. Then insert a pencil or screwdriver into the bandage, on the side of the wound nearest the heart. Twist the tourniquet until the bleeding stops.

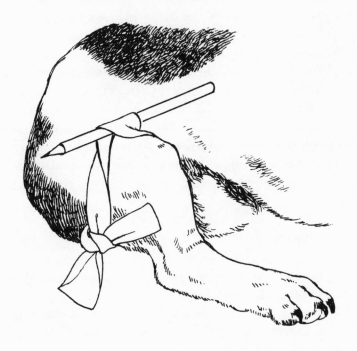

Venous wounds: Blood flowing from a vein flows regularly, rather than being pumped out. The color is dark red.

Treatment: For venous wounds, apply the tourniquet *below* the wound and twist until the bleeding stops. Keep the tourniquet tight for no more than one minute. Then loosen slightly. Every ten minutes loosen the tourniquet completely to see if the bleeding has stopped, and to allow the blood to reach the rest of the leg and prevent tissue damage.

Transportation of Injured Dogs

General: If an injured dog must be moved, before you do anything, know exactly what you are going to do. Before you move the injured animal, decide where you are going to move it. A little foresight can save a lot of agony. Remember, a dog in pain will attempt to bite and scratch. Be careful when you approach the dog. (See Restraint and Handling.)

Before you move an injured dog: Tie its jaws closed. If the dog is bleeding profusely, stop the *bleeding* before moving the animal. Check for a possible fractured spine by pinching between the injured animal's toes. If it does not register pain, there is a strong possibility that the spine is broken. In this event, do not move the dog unless it is lying in the middle of a road.

Technique for moving injured dogs: Small dogs may be lifted by the scruff of the neck and carried to your car. If there is someone with you, have him hold the injured dog while you drive. If you are alone, place the injured dog on the floor of the car, in the front, on the passenger side. Larger dogs will require a stretcher or sling of some sort. A blanket, coat, or the back seat of the car will serve. Both large and small dogs should be covered with a blanket or coat. This will help to minimize the danger of *shock*, by keeping the dog warm as well as providing a degree of restraint. Do not give the injured dog anything to drink: no tea, no water, no alcohol. This is to prevent vomiting if an anesthetic has to be administered.

Vaccination

A vaccine is an injection of a preparation of living or dead viruses that provides immunity to certain viral or bacterial diseases.

Natural immunity: Puppies receive antibodies from the mother's first milk (colostrum). This provides a natural immunity that lasts for eight to ten weeks and then diminishes. In order not to interfere with this natural immunity, puppies are usually not vaccinated until they are ten weeks old.

Orphan puppies: Orphan puppies, which are being fed on supplements and have not received colostrum, should be given an injection (by a vet) of either gamma globulin or a live vaccine when they are two days old. They should be vaccinated at eight weeks and again at twelve and sixteen weeks of age, to insure a high immunity against distemper and hepatitis.

Dog vaccines: A single combination vaccine is available to prevent distemper (hard pad), hepatitis, the two types of leptospirosis, and rabies.

Weaning

Weaning is the process of taking a puppy off its mother's milk and putting it on a diet of more adult food.

Puppies begin showing an interest in solid foods at three or four weeks of age. This does not mean that they are quite ready to be weaned. But their interest should be encouraged by offering them small amounts of finely chopped meat, deboned fish or chicken, and bowls of milk, three or four times a day.

When the puppies are four to five weeks old they are ready to be weaned. By the time the mother begins vomiting her food (soft, partially digested) for her youngsters to eat, they should be completely weaned.

At about eight weeks of age, recently weaned puppies should be given five meals a day: three of meat (either fresh or canned food), and two of cereal (i.e., fine puppy meal, cornflakes, or farina mixed with milk). If you wish, commercial dry food preparations may be given. With dry foods, feed up to five times a day, depending on the breed.

2

Problems of the Head and Neck

THE EAR

Acute Middle Ear Infection

Cause: Usually seen as the sequel to simple ear complaints which have not been treated.

Symptoms: Loss of balance. The dog may walk around with its head constantly on one side, or it may have difficulty in standing.

Treatment: This condition is an emergency. The infection can spread rapidly to the brain, causing severe meningitis, encephalitis, and death. Antibiotics must be administered as soon as possible. Get professional assistance.

Acute Otitis (See also Ear Mites)

Symptoms: Often occurs after ear mite infection. Symptoms may be similar to those of ear mites, but with severe inflammation. This condition is caused by a bacterial infection and treatment must be given by a professional.

Home Treatment: To relieve the acute itching and soreness, pour warm olive oil into the ear. To relieve discomfort, administer one 5-grain aspirin tablet per 20 pounds of body weight, up to 25 grains, once a day. (See How to Administer Tablets and Pills.) Remember that these are only temporary measures to be used until professional help is available. Acute otitis cannot be cured at home.

Warning: If left untreated, this condition can develop into a middle ear infection.

Bleeding or Hemorrhaging from the Ear

Often seen after fights or road accidents. Bleeding may be from the earflap or from inside the ear.

Treatment: Whether the bleeding originates from the earflap or from the ear itself, the treatment is the same. Pack the ear canal with absorbent cotton (just enough to fill the ear without overpacking). Bandage the ear. (See Bandaging the Ear.) The bandage may be left on for three to four days.

Warning: If left untreated, bleeding from the ear may develop into a middle ear infection.

Blood Blister on the Ear (Hematoma)

A thick, fluctuating, irregular swelling usually found inside the earflap, but the outside may also be involved. The blister itself is painless and firmer than an abscess.

Causes: These blisters come up quite suddenly, usually

as the result of a blow, a bite, as the sequel to an ear mite infestation, or from an irritation which causes constant scratching. Such an irritation might be caused by an infection in the ear, in which case it will be accompanied by pus coming from the ear canal.

Treatment: If the blister is the result of an ear infection and is small, leave it alone and treat the infection. (See Acute Middle Ear Infection.) If the blood blister is not the result of an infection, just bandage it. Quite often the bandaging will cause the blister to be absorbed naturally.

Technique: Wrap the bandage around the ear, then bandage the ear to the head.

Treatment for persistent blister: If the blister has not disappeared after being bandaged for three or four days, and if it is fairly small (about an inch in diameter), you can drain it yourself. Sterilize a needle by boiling it for twenty minutes. Wash your hands. Prick the blister on the inside of the earflap with the sterile needle and allow it to drain naturally. *(Do not squeeze it.)* After the blister drains, bandage the ear to prevent infection and further irritation. With larger blisters (more than an inch in diameter), it is advisable to seek professional assistance.

Blood blisters (hematomas), while not serious in themselves, can easily cause permanent disfigurement of the ear. The best first aid is to keep them bandaged and taped to the dog's head to prevent the animal from scratching them and making them worse. If the dog persists in scratching, use an Elizabethan collar to discourage him. (See Elizabethan Collar.)

Deafness

Deafness may be either hereditary or acquired.

Hereditary deafness: Usually seen in white dogs with blue eyes. Dogs suffering from hereditary deafness should be neutered to prevent them from passing on the condition.

Acquired deafness: Acquired deafness often occurs as the result of ear infections or accidents. It may be temporary or irreversible, depending upon the cause and severity of the condition.

Partial deafness: Partial deafness occurs in elderly dogs, and in younger ones that have ingested lead poisons.

Symptoms: Deaf animals may appear to be stupid, do not respond to their names or to commands, and bark continually. A definite diagnosis of true deafness is difficult, since the deaf dog is compensated by the enhancement of its other sensory perceptions, especially its ability to detect vibrations.

Ear Mites (Otodectic Mange)

Symptoms: There is acute irritation of the ears and the dog spends much time scratching its ears and shaking its head. Brown, waxy discharge, containing crusts, can be seen in the ears. There may be a rattling noise from the ears when the dog shakes its head.

Treatment: In the early stages, clean the dog's ears with absorbent cotton dipped in a very dilute mixture of mild liquid detergent (1 teaspoon detergent liquid to ½ cup water). This will get rid of the sticky wax.

Be careful when cleaning the ears, but you need not be

afraid of touching the eardrum since it is well out of the way of the cotton. Do not use a cotton bud or Q-tip ®. This may damage the eardrum. After cleaning, swab the inside with a solution containing rotenone (e. g., Canolene ®) once a week for a month. This solution is available from veterinarians. More acute cases may require professional treatment.

Foreign Bodies in the Ear

Symptoms: Excessive shaking of the head; scratching of the ear.

Treatment: Most foreign bodies in the ear can be removed by pouring a little olive oil or cooking oil into the ear, then gently massaging it until the object is floated out.

Warning: Do not poke anything smaller than your left elbow into the dog's ear. If you cannot remove the object by the olive oil method, take the dog to a vet. (See Acute Otitis.)

THE EYE

Blindness

Sudden blindness: The result of either a stroke or an accident in which the dog's brain or eyes have been injured.

Temporary blindness: Occurs during infections of the cornea (clear part of the eye), (e.g., keratitis). These infections are accompanied by acute pain, crying, tearing, and extreme sensitivity to light. If not properly treated by a professional, these infections can give rise to milkiness and eventually to ulceration of the cornea.

If corneal ulcer occurs, immediate professional treatment is vital. Do not bathe the eye; this may cause the ulcer to rupture. Corneal ulcers take a long time to heal, and the dog may be left with a black scar on the cornea. The condition frequently occurs in breeds with bulbous eyes (e.g., Pekingese and pugs).

Progressive blindness: This common condition is usually the result of old age causing the formation of cataracts. These cataracts can also be caused by diabetes mellitus. (See Diabetes Mellitus.)

Treatment: If you suspect that your dog is going blind, and the symptoms are painfully obvious—bumping into things, unable to recognize people at a distance, etc.—have the animal examined by a vet. He will be able to make a definite diagnosis and possibly treat with enzyme injections, or in the case of cataracts, by surgery.

If the condition is irreversible, the dog owner should be aware that blindness need not mean the end of the animal's life. When the eyes fail, the other senses develop to compensate. Blind animals, as a rule, hear and smell much better than sighted animals. By the time the dog is completely blind, it will know its way around the house, and be able to go for walks on a leash. Blind animals, on the whole, manage remarkably well. They need just a little extra care. Most dogs, even those with normal eyesight, do not really see very well. In addition, most dogs are color-blind.

Brown Stains in the Corner of the Eye

Certain breeds, especially the poodle, may develop brown staining in the corner of the eye.

Cause: Blockage or absence of tear ducts; weeping.

Treatment: Prepare a dilute solution of hydrogen peroxide: 1 teaspoon hydrogen peroxide to 10 teaspoons water; and bathe the stains liberally. Do not bathe the eyeball, only the stains. This not only gets rid of the stains, but it may also remove the obstruction in blockage of the tear ducts.

Cataract

A cataract is an opacity and hardening of the lens of the eye that prevents light from passing through.

Causes: The most common cause of cataracts is old age. Keep in mind that cataracts cause varying degrees of blindness. In an elderly dog, the lens may appear quite opaque and yet a certain amount of vision is still possible.

If cataracts appear in the eyes of younger dogs, a disease state such as diabetes must be considered.

Symptoms: A gradual, growing opacity or milkiness of the pupil.

Treatment: Cataracts, like every serious eye condition, must be treated by a professional. This treatment should begin as soon as the dog owner notices the cloudiness. Delay can prevent possible cure.

If the cataracts are caused by diabetes, professional treatment of the disease may halt the growth of the cataracts. If old age is the cause, the vet may suggest waiting until the cataract ripens, and then operating on it.

In many cases, a nonfunctional lens can be surgically removed, resulting in the return of a fair degree of vision.

Conjunctivitis and Other Infectious Eye Conditions

Although it is not contagious to humans, conjunctivitis can be transmitted to other animals. Quarantine the infected dog.

Symptoms: The affected eye reddens and is sore to the touch. A sticky, yellowish discharge is exuded from the eye. The eye hurts and the dog continually rubs its face on the ground.

Treatment: Prepare a saline solution: boil 1 pint of water, add 1 teaspoon of table salt, and allow the solution to cool. Bathe the eye liberally with the solution every two hours for the next twenty-four hours. Soak a wad of absorbent cotton in the saline solution and then squeeze the cotton so that the solution floods the dog's eye.

If the condition has not cleared up after thirty-six hours, consult a vet. (See Foreign Bodies in the Eye.) Proprietary eye ointments, often sold in pet shops, are *not* recommended.

Eyeball out of Socket

This sometimes occurs after fights or highway accidents, particularly in certain breeds with bulbous eyes (e.g., Pekingese, King Charles spaniel, bulldog).

Treatment: Apply olive oil or Vaseline ® to the eye socket and gently try to ease the eyeball back into place. Then bandage over.

If the eyeball will not fit, or will not stay in the eye socket, hold the eye in place with damp or oily absorbent cotton. (Saturate cotton with olive oil.) Bandage over lightly. (See Bandaging the Eye.) Get professional help.

Foreign Bodies in the Eye

The foreign body may be a grass seed, a sliver of glass, a bit of grit, a grain of sand, or anything else that doesn't belong in the eye.

If the foreign body perforates the eyeball, it will cause extreme pain. Do not attempt to remove an object that has punctured the eyeball. Get the dog to a vet at once.

Symptoms: Sudden and profuse tearing, but the tears flow out of one eye only. There will be acute irritation of that eyeball as well.

Treatment: Make a sterile saline solution by adding 1 teaspoon table salt to 1 pint water. Bring the water to a boil. Allow time for the water to cool. Bathe the eye liberally with this solution, using an eyedropper, or a wad of cotton saturated with the solution and squeezed into the eye. Apply a soothing ophthalmic ointment (consult your pharmacist) directly onto the eyeball.

The technique for applying the ointment is to place the thumb and index finger of the left hand above and below the affected eye. Squeeze the ointment into the corner of the eye with your right hand. Close the eyelid with the thumb and index finger of your left hand and hold it closed for a few seconds. This will spread the ointment over the whole eyeball.

If the dog persists in scratching after the treatment, the foreign body may still be in the eye. Take the dog to the vet.

One of the most common causes of foreign objects in the eye is the result of dogs leaning their heads out of car windows. Exposure of the eyes to high winds can be injurious, so roll up the window when you take your dog for a car ride.

Glaucoma (Swelling of the Eye)

Causes: This condition is caused by failure of the fluid in the eye to circulate properly, causing pressure to build up inside the eye. Often a breed failure, glaucoma is commonly seen in wire-haired fox terriers, bull terriers, cocker spaniels and bassets.

Symptoms: The eyeball increases in size and protrudes from the eye socket. There is associated conjunctivitis and, in later stages, corneal opacity (a cloudiness of the front of the eye).

Treatment: Glaucoma, like all eye conditions, must be treated by a professional. A vet will administer drugs to improve the circulation of fluid.

THE MOUTH

Teething Stages in Puppies

Like humans, dogs have two sets of teeth. The temporary teeth (baby teeth) appear about three weeks after birth. These are replaced by the permanent teeth, which appear from five months onward. As the permanent teeth push through the gums, they displace the temporary teeth, which are either spit out or swallowed. By six to seven months of age, all the permanent teeth are in. Dogs have twenty-eight temporary teeth and forty-two permanent teeth.

Complications: The temporary canine teeth often remain in the dog's mouth after the secondary or permanent teeth have appeared. These extra teeth may have to be extracted when the dog is six to eight months old. This condition is common in the smaller breeds, especially the Yorkie, the poodle, and the dachshund.

Care of teeth: Dogs should have regular dental checkups by a vet, to prevent gingivitis, periodontitis, halitosis, and eventual tooth loss. The wise owner will accustom his dog to having its teeth cleaned regularly with toothpaste or with a mild tooth powder on moist absorbent cotton.

Bad Breath (Halitosis)

As a general rule, a dog with bad breath is not well. If the condition persists for more than forty-eight hours, seek professional advice.

Causes: In dogs under six months of age, bad breath sometimes accompanies teething. It also may indicate a worm infestation. In older animals, bad breath may indicate a number of diseases: tonsillitis, stomach infection, stomatitis (an ulcer of the mouth), infected or broken teeth, labial eczema (a condition of the lips, fairly common in spaniels), or sinusitis.

With elderly dogs, continuing halitosis may indicate a degree of chronic kidney failure.

Treatment: First, insofar as possible, check for disease states. Does the dog "act" sick? Is it feverish? Apathetic? Once these disease states have been eliminated as possible causes for bad breath, treat the condition by administering chlorophyll tablets or charcoal tablets. Dosage: one to six tablets a day, depending upon size (one tablet per 10 pounds of body weight, up to six tablets a day). (See How to Administer Tablets and Pills.)

Broken Tooth

Occasionally, a dog breaks a tooth by biting too hard on something harder than its tooth.

This is not an emergency, although the broken tooth may have to be extracted eventually. Very cold or very hard substances may further damage the exposed part of the tooth.

Symptoms: Drooling, slight bleeding from the mouth; bad breath.

Gingivitis

Gingivitis is an infection of the gums which appears at the margin of tooth and gum.

Cause: It is often seen in association with tartar.

Symptoms: The classic symptom of this infection is a narrow red line along the gum, above the tooth or teeth. The animal also has halitosis.

Treatment: Since gingivitis is often caused by general

infections of the mouth and throat as well as by more specific infections, the exact cause of the condition must be identified and eliminated.

Gingivitis is easily treated by applying a solution made from hydrogen peroxide. Use 1 part hydrogen peroxide to 3 parts water. Alternatively, a solution of 1 part tincture of iodine to 30 parts glycerin may be used.

Swab the gums with this solution every three hours. If the condition has not cleared up after three days of treatment, seek professional help.

Specific Abscess: Tooth Root or Molar Abscess

The "specific" abscess is found on the upper tooth roots.
Cause: Decayed tooth.

Symptoms: If an abcess constantly recurs below the dog's eye or along the line of the jaw, examine the dog's mouth. A decayed tooth may be causing the abscess. The abscess itself is a pus-discharging sore that appears on the dog's face. (See Abscesses.)

Treatment: There is no home treatment for this condition. Tooth root abscesses require extraction of the tooth and antibiotic treatment. Consult a vet.

Tartar on the Teeth

Causes: All dogs living in hard water areas eventually develop tartar on their teeth. Tartar and periodontitis (an infection of the gums) may be related, especially in older dogs, to chronic kidney failure.

Symptoms: Bad breath (halitosis); excessive salivation;

pawing and rubbing at the mouth. While obviously hungry, the dog either refuses to eat, or begins to eat, then spits out the food.

Should these symptoms occur, examine your dog's teeth. Tartar looks like brown crusts on the teeth.

Treatment: In the early stages tartar can be rubbed off with smoker's tooth powder (a mild, abrasive tooth powder available at drugstores). In particularly stubborn cases, professional scaling by a vet may be necessary.

Prevention: Prevention of tartar accumulation can be accomplished by regular (once a month) cleaning of the dog's teeth with either ordinary toothpaste or absorbent cotton, or with smoker's tooth powder on moist absorbent cotton. The wise owner will avoid a good deal of trouble by getting the dog accustomed to regular tooth brushings.

THE TONGUE

Bitten Tongue

This is a common condition in dogs and can be very serious.

Symptoms: Profuse bleeding from the mouth.

Treatment: A bitten tongue may sound like a minor mishap, but if the bleeding is very heavy it is an emergency. Since the tongue is constantly moist and moving, it is difficult for a blood clot to form, so that bleeding is continuous. If the cut is deep enough, the dog can bleed to death. Fortunately, it would take several hours, at the least, for this to happen, which gives you plenty of time to get the dog to a vet. If the dog will allow it, hold its tongue in a cotton pad to reduce the bleeding, while you are transporting the animal to the vet.

Inflammation of the Tongue (Glossitis)

Causes: Numerous; most of them serious. The inflammation could be the result of chronic interstitial nephritis, corrosive poisons, fishhooks, or other trauma.

Symptoms: Severe dribbling, accompanied by loss of appetite and halitosis. Open the dog's mouth and look for raw, red, sore patches. (See How to Open a Dog's Mouth.) These are ulcers on the tongue. In later stages there is a foul, brownish drainage from the corner of the mouth that drips down the chest and paws. Look for drainage stains on the dog's chest and paws.

Treatment: The dog's mouth must be kept as clean as possible by washing it with a solution of 3% hydrogen peroxide: add 1 teaspoon 3% hydrogen peroxide to 1 pint water. Administer the solution every two hours. If there is no improvement after twenty-four hours contact a vet.

THE NOSE

Nasal Discharge

A thick, yellowish mucus discharge suggests distemper or one of the other canine virus diseases. (See Sinusitis.)

Normally, a healthy dog's nose is cold and wet. A hot, dry nose suggests fever and warrants further investigation. Consult a vet.

Nosebleed (Epistaxis)

Nosebleeds are symptoms, and the dog owner should be more concerned with the cause than with the nosebleed itself. In most instances a nosebleed will subside of its own accord fairly quickly.

Causes: Nosebleeds can be the result of car accidents; a sharp blow; tumors; decayed tooth sockets; excessive sneezing; foreign bodies in the nose; high blood pressure; or minute parasites in the nose.

Treatment: Sponge the nostrils dry with absorbent cotton. Examine the nostrils under a good light to determine the cause or site of the hemorrhage.

If your dog is calm and has been well trained, you should be able to do this yourself; otherwise, you may need an assistant. (See Restraint and Handling.) If you can see a foreign body, and if the dog remains calm, you may be able to remove it with tweezers. If you cannot see anything, do not poke about in the animal's nostrils. The mucous membrane that lines the nostrils is very sensitive and easily injured.

If the cause of the nosebleed is not apparent, keep the dog as still as possible. Apply cold compresses or ice cubes to the bridge of the nose. Do not stuff or pack the nostrils. This will cause the dog to sneeze and make the bleeding worse.

Tip of the nose: Bleeding from the tip of the nose can be persistent and, if too much blood is lost, potentially dangerous. It can be controlled by pressure with the fingers. (See illustration on page 82.)

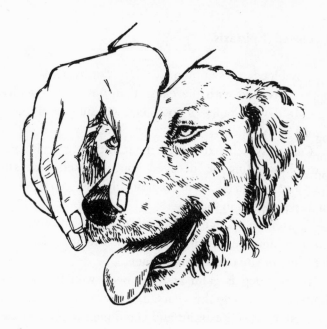

Sinusitis

Sinusitis is an infection of the sinuses. (The sinuses are an extension of the nasal chamber, located in the front of the dog's head.)

Causes: The infection may be caused either by germs or by a foreign body in the nose.

Symptoms: Except in the case of foreign bodies, sinusitis rarely occurs on its own. Usually it is seen as a sequel to viral conditions such as distemper. The symptoms themselves are: a yellowish nasal discharge; bouts of sneezing; and loss of appetite.

Treatment: Since many other illnesses are characterized by the same symptoms, you will need professional help to make a definite diagnosis. If the symptoms continue for more than twenty-four hours, take the dog to a vet. If it is sinusitis, the vet will probably administer a course of antibiotics.

If a vet is not immediately available, home treatment consists of: keeping the dog's face clean of the mucous discharge, and assisting the dog to breathe normally by clearing its nasal passages. This is accomplished by having the dog inhale a preparation of menthol (available at drugstores) in hot water. To make this preparation, pour some boiling water into a large, shallow tin dish (a pie tin) and add 3 tablespoons menthol to the boiling water. Then, calmly but firmly, hold the dog's face over the steam for a moment or two.

Try to treat this inhalation as an ordinary occurrence. The trick is to have the dog inhale as much of the vapor as possible; this is only effective if the dog is not alarmed. Also, you do not want to hold a struggling frightened dog over boiling water, so do not force your pet. Handle the animal with confidence.

Sneezing

Continual sneezing is a much more serious symptom in dogs than in people.

Intermittent sneezing: If the dog sneezes on and off for a few hours, but seems all right otherwise—no fever, no apathy, etc.—the sneezing is probably due to simple irritation, such as dust up its nose.

Prolonged sneezing: If the dog continues to sneeze throughout the day, refuses food, and there is an accompanying nasal discharge, suspect an infection and get professional assistance.

Bouts of strenuous sneezing: Strenuous and continued sneezing suggests a foreign body in the nose.

Examine the nostrils with a flashlight. If the foreign object is visible, use tweezers and remove it carefully.

Warning: If you do not see anything, don't poke about with the tweezers. The nasal lining is easily ruptured. (See Nosebleed.)

THE THROAT

Choking

Choking takes place when either the tongue or a foreign body blocks the back of the throat and prevents the dog from breathing. Choking often looks worse than it really is because the dog panics, which makes it choke even more, which makes it panic even more... Don't you panic too.

Treatment: If the dog has fainted (from lack of oxygen), open its mouth and pull its tongue out. Make certain that nothing is blocking the windpipe. If there is an obstruction, do not try to push whatever it is down the throat. Hook it out with your finger. Once the throat is clear, if the dog is still unconscious, administer artificial respiration.

If the dog is conscious, hold it upside down by its hind legs and thump it on the back. This may dislodge whatever is at the back of its throat. If it does not, and the dog is still choking, open its mouth (see Restraint and Handling), and use your fingers to fish out the foreign object. If the object is stuck, pour a little olive oil down the animal's throat to lubricate the gullet. If your probing causes the dog to gag, so much the better, as this may bring up the obstruction.

Hopefully, there is no need to worry about being bitten;

with your hand down the dog's throat, the animal will be too busy trying to breathe to bite the hand that is trying to save it.

Prevention: Dogs often choke on small, hard rubber balls that are given to them to play with. These are difficult to dislodge from the throat and should be avoided. The softer, hollow type of ball is much safer.

Bones that lodge sideways in the animal's throat are a common cause of choking. This can be prevented by not feeding the dog bones. They are not necessary for your pet's well-being.

Fishhooks

If a dog gets a fishhook caught in its mouth or anywhere on its body, take it to a vet at once. It is simple to remove a fishhook after the dog has had a general anesthetic. Unfortunately, most fishhook accidents happen in places remote from vets and it may be up to you to remove the hook.

Preparation procedure: Get someone to hold the dog. It is almost impossible to hold the animal and operate at the same time. So even if it takes a little longer, find someone to assist you. You will need: the best light you can get; a pair of needle-nosed pincers or wire-cutters; a sharp knife or a razor blade (boil it for twenty minutes).

Assuming the hook is not caught in the mouth, slip a tape muzzle over the animal's mouth and have your assistant hold the dog under a good light. (See Restraint and Handling.) If the hook is caught in the mouth, the assistant will hold the mouth open. You are now ready to remove the hook.

Operative procedure: Think about what you are doing

before you do anything. Examine the way the hook is embedded. Do not try to pull the hook out, or you will tear a huge, bleeding chunk out of the dog. Determine which way the barb is pointing and push it out through the skin. Use the pincers or wire cutters to snip off the head of the hook. Then pull the hook out. (Pull in the opposite direction from where the barb was pointing.)

If the hook is embedded in a way that prevents you from getting at the head, use the sharp, sterile knife to make an incision over the area where the head of the hook is embedded. Don't be squeamish. Your incision will do a lot less damage than a forceful pull. After you have made the incision, use the pincers to snip off the head of the hook.

Dress the wound to prevent infection (see Wounds), unless the hook has been removed from mouth or throat, in which case no dressing is necessary.

Swallowing Safety Pins or Other Sharp Objects

Feed the dog bread or porridge. Also feed it small balls of absorbent cotton which have been dipped in meat extract or meat flavoring. Avoid force-feeding.

Then get professional advice. It may be necessary to X-ray the animal.

Tonsillitis and Foreign Bodies in the Throat

These conditions produce similar symptoms.

General symptoms: The dog coughs, licks its lips, appears distressed, and may cry out in pain. It refuses food and may appear apathetic or sleepy.

Bones stuck between the larynx and the stomach cause no loss of appetite, but the dog vomits when it eats. There is also excessive dribbling and profound depression. There is no home treatment for bones lodged in this area. Consult a vet.

Tonsillitis symptoms: The dog will be retching, coughing, licking its lips. The dog is depressed and lethargic and has a high fever (over 103°F.). (See Taking Temperature.) When you open the dog's mouth, the tonsils, which are at the back of the throat, will look like two swollen, strawberry-colored lumps.

Treatment: Calm the dog with petting and soothing words. Then administer one or two aspirin tablets per day, depending on the size of the dog. Give no food or water, except for some cracked ice, until a vet has examined the dog. Put the ice into a perforated bowl (a soap dish with holes punched into it is ideal), so that the dog can moisten its mouth by licking the ice but cannot drink.

Foreign body in the throat or mouth: First, open the dog's mouth. Using a flashlight, look down its throat. (See How to Open a Dog's Mouth.) If there is a foreign body such as a bone stuck in the dog's throat, use your fingers or, if it is too far down to reach, a pair of needlenosed pliers, to work it out. Do not jerk it out or you may tear the lining of the throat.

3

Problems of the Skin and Hair

THE SKIN

Skin Diseases: General

Dogs can develop acute skin conditions very quickly. These painful, unhealthy conditions should not be allowed to continue. Prompt treatment by the dog owner can prevent nuisances from becoming serious problems.

The most obvious indication of skin problems is excessive scratching. Any dog that is continually scratching itself either has trouble or is headed for trouble. The owner must take note of this scratching and set about discovering its cause.

Skin diseases have a public health aspect. Some, such as ringworm and sarcoptic mange, can be transmitted from animals to people. Others (e.g., demodectic mange), are transmitted from animal to animal.

Skin diseases take various forms and many factors are

involved, but for purposes of home treatment, we can divide skin diseases into: (1) Contagious (transmitted by direct contact). (2) Infectious (transmitted through the air), such as ringworm. (3) Noncontagious and noninfectious, such as eczema and diseases caused by hormonal imbalance.

Contagious: Contagious diseases such as mange or ringworm should be treated under strict hygienic conditions, and the affected dog should be kept away from other animals and from small children.

Noncontagious: With noncontagious skin diseases, the owner may not feel the same urgency for treatment. Some owners, in time, even "learn to live with" their dog's condition. These owners would do better to learn to cure it. Aside from eventual worsening of the original complaint, neglect invites a host of secondary complications. All abnormal skin conditions should be diagnosed and treated at once.

In the noncontagious category of skin diseases, perhaps the most common is warts. These may be due to viruses, but this has not been proved.

If the owner will take his dog to a vet when he first observes this growth, it is usually simple to remove. The longer the owner waits, the more difficult and dangerous the operation becomes.

Hormonal imbalance: This is a common cause of noncontagious skin disease. The imbalance can produce bald spots as well as certain varieties of eczema. If the symptoms are observed and treatment instituted early, the condition can be corrected quickly.

Hereditary diseases: Owners of highly bred dogs, especially those bred for certain abnormal traits, such as the folds and protruding eyes of the bulldog and the squashed nose of the Peke, should be aware of the particular skin diseases their animal's breeding makes it heir to (e.g., spaniels, labial eczema; dachshunds, frictional dermatitis of the armpit).

Neuroses: High-strung dogs and dogs which need a lot of exercise and are not getting it, or dogs which are simply neurotic (yes, there are such creatures) may develop skin diseases by continuously licking themselves. Usually they pick out a spot on their foreleg and lick it until the skin breaks.

Treatment: Apply calamine lotion to the affected spot. If the dog continues to chew and lick at it, it may be necessary to bandage the area. An Elizabethan collar may also be useful. (See Elizabethan Collar.)

External origins: Chemicals, accidents, foreign bodies (such as grass seeds), even overexposure to light, can cause a skin disease.

Allergies: Probably the most common of noncontagious skin diseases are those caused by allergies. Unfortunately, they are also the most difficult to cure.

Abscesses

An abscess is a swelling caused by a collection of pus under the dog's skin. This swelling is accompanied by localized pain and heat.

Normally, the swelling grows larger and larger until "pointing" occurs. When this happens, the abscess softens and finally bursts.

Treatment: Encourage the abscess to point by: bathing it in hot saline solution, and applying hot compresses directly over the abscess until it bursts. When it does burst, wash away the pus with a solution of 2 teaspoons of 3% hydrogen peroxide added to 1 pint warm water.

With abscesses that do not drain completely, bathe every two hours with warm saltwater, to keep the abscess open and draining (1 teaspoon table salt to 1 pint warm water).

Warning: Do not squeeze an abscess. Allow it to burst naturally. An abscess is formed by the body in order to wall off an infection. When you squeeze the abscess, you are breaking down the wall and forcing the infection back into the body.

Bites and Fight Wounds

There are two types of wounds received from animal bites: puncture wounds and lacerated wounds.

Puncture wounds: These are small, deep holes in the skin, often accompanied by bruising. Puncture wounds are the most serious kind of bite wounds and are usually infected. If a puncture wound is left untreated, the skin will heal but an abscess will form underneath.

Treatment: Clean the area around the wound with soap and water, or a 10% solution of hydrogen peroxide. Since puncture wounds are nearly always infected, antibiotics, which require a prescription, should be given by a vet.

Lacerated wounds: The wound is jagged, the skin is torn, and there may be profuse bleeding.

Treatment: Clean the wound with hydrogen peroxide or soap and water. Check to be sure that the wound has drained and that there is no infection left. If the wound is discharging pus, it is still infected. If the wound is very large, it may require stitches. Consult a vet.

Capped Elbow

A common condition in larger dogs: Alsatians, Great Danes, mastiffs, and St. Bernards.

Cause: Lying on hard floors. Because of the dog's great weight, its skin is damaged and a protective reaction, the capped elbow, occurs.

Symptoms: A fluctuating, fluid-filled swelling develops at the elbow. The hair around the swelling falls out and the skin thickens. Open sores (ulcerations) may develop. In later stages, the swelling becomes hard and fibrous.

Treatment: During the early stages of the swelling, apply cold compresses to the swelling. Although a capped elbow is not an emergency, it should not be ignored. If you let it go for too long, surgical drainage and dissection may be necessary.

Preventive measures: If you have a large dog, make sure that it has a soft bed to lie on.

Fleas

Fleas, like taxes, are a perennial problem for dog owners. Fleas not only cause your dog intense irritation and discomfort, they also carry tapeworm eggs. Your dog's fleas may bite you, but you will be glad to know that it is only in passing; dog fleas will not live on humans.

Symptoms: When grooming your dog, if you notice small, reddish, flat creatures running through the hair, your dog has fleas. When the hair of a dog with fleas is parted, it will look as if tiny particles of black grit have been scattered through the hairs. These are flea droppings.

Treatment: Bathe the dog with a shampoo containing selenium sulfide (available at drugstores) every three days for two weeks. On the days when the dog is not being bathed, powder it thoroughly with rotenone powder or pyrethrum powder (available at drugstores and most pet stores). During the flea season, which varies with locale, the dog should wear a flea collar (available at pet stores). Change the collar at regular intervals of three to five weeks. Supplement baths and powderings with patented aerosol sprays, which kill fleas on contact (available at pet stores). Dust liberal amounts of flea powder on and around the dog's sleeping areas.

Treatment for puppies: Puppies under eight weeks of age should not be powdered. Simply bathe them in a diluted selenium sulfide shampoo. Make sure that you wash off all the shampoo after bathing. Dry them well.

While defleaing the dog, be sure that the dog's environment, your home, is free of fleas. To remove fleas from carpets and cushions, spray with any patented fly-killing aerosol available at hardware stores. For heavy infestation, call an exterminator.

Lice

Lice are flat gray, wingless insects, sometimes confused with fleas. But fleas can be seen running through the dog's hair, while lice crawl slowly, or cling to the base of the hairs.

Although animal lice will not live on humans for very

long, they carry disease and cause intense irritation to dogs that may lead to complications and must not be neglected.

Treatment: Shampoo and bathe the dog twice a week for two weeks with a shampoo containing selenium sulfide (e.g., Seleen ®), with gamma-benzene hexachloride washes (an insecticide, available at drugstores).

In addition to the biweekly shampoo, apply a flea powder containing rotenone (available at drugstores) over the whole dog once a week.

Caution: When treating puppies (under six months), just use the shampoo once a week. Avoid flea powders, as they may be toxic to young dogs.

Mange

Mange is a common parasitic skin disease caused by microscopic spiderlike mites.

General symptoms: You will observe your dog's discomfort: it will bite and scratch at the infested areas. There is also loss of hair, reddening of the skin and, occasionally, thickening of the skin.

There are two types of mange which affect dogs: demodectic mange (sometimes called "follicular" or "red" mange) and sarcoptic mange, which is contagious to people.

Demodectic and sarcoptic mange have some general symptoms in common, but only a microscopic examination of the skin scrapings can produce a definite diagnosis; since the treatment depends upon whether the mange is demodectic or sarcoptic, you have to be certain. There are two ways to deal with this problem. You can take the dog to a vet, who will take a skin scraping. Or you can give general treatment which is effective in both cases.

General treatment: Bathe the entire animal in warm water with gamma benzene hexachloride powder added (available at drugstores): use 8 ounces powder to 1 gallon water. Or, use a selenium sulfide shampoo (e.g., Seleen ®). Repeat this bath every five days. In most cases, three or four baths will be enough to cure the mange. Provide relief from excessive biting and scratching, as this can cause secondary infections and other unpleasant complications. If the animal will not stop biting itself, fit it with an Elizabethan collar. You may also provide temporary relief by applying a soothing, cooling lotion (e.g., calamine lotion) to the irritated areas.

Dispose of the dog's bedding. Use an undiluted solution of pHisoDerm ® to wash the dog's collar or harness, twice a week for as long as the condition persists. Do not allow your dog to come into contact with other animals. When you walk the dog, keep it on the leash.

After every treatment, use liberal amounts of soap, water, and pHisoDerm ® to thoroughly clean and disinfect the area where you have been treating the dog. Dispose of the absorbent cotton where no one will handle it. Then wash your own hands.

Warning: Never use carbolic soap or Lysol ® to wash your dog. Dogs absorb the carbolic and Lysol ® through their skin and though these preparations will kill the dog's mange, they may also kill the dog.

Ringworm

Ringworm is a disease of the the top layer of the skin (epidermis) caused by two groups of fungi, both of which are contagious and infectious and can affect human beings. Ringworm is rare in dogs and easily confused with other skin diseases, such as demodectic mange.

Symptoms: Breaks in the skin appear on the head and chest. These are dry, scaly patches, circular in shape, up to an inch across in diameter. These lesions vary from very slight to scaling of the skin, followed by a pus-forming infection.

Treatment: Clip the hair around the breaks in the skin. Apply a solution of benzyl-benzoate to the lesions and the surrounding area. Saturate absorbent cotton in the solution and continue application once a day for as long as the breaks in the skin are visible. The most successful treatment for ringworm is the oral administration of griseofulvin tablets. Always wash your hands after treating a dog with ringworm.

In healthy dogs, the condition may disappear spontaneously, in about two months. But do not wait two months, because in addition to being contagious, ringworm is a highly unpleasant and very uncomfortable disease and should be treated at the first sign.

Sebaceous Cyst

Cause: Blockage of the duct of a sweat gland.
Description: These cysts are found on the dog's skin,

usually on its back. They often have a pustular head and resemble a miniature volcano.

Treatment: If you leave the cyst alone, it will usually rise to a head and eventually pop, discharging a cheesy substance.

When the cyst does pop, it should be thoroughly squeezed out. The area around the cyst should be bathed with a dilute solution of pHisoDerm ® and water (1 teaspoon to 10 teaspoons water).

Occasionally, a sebaceous cyst will rise to a head, pop, and continue to discharge without healing. If the cyst does not stop discharging, it will require surgical removal.

Ticks

The tick is a blood-sucking parasite with a shiny spherical body, varying in size from one-quarter to one-half inch in diameter. The tick is creamy gray in color, and looks like a soybean with tiny legs at one end.

Country animals often come into contact with the common sheep tick. Usually, ticks are first noticed when you are grooming your dog. Another good reason for frequent grooming.

Treatment: Do not try to pull the tick out. Ticks have powerful sucking jaws that burrow into the dog's skin. If you try to pull the tick out, its head will break off, leaving the mouth of the tick under the dog's skin, and a sinus may eventually form. (A sinus is a discharging wound that does not heal.) The trick is to get the tick to remove its mouth before you pull it off your dog. There are three techniques for accomplishing this:

(1) Pour a little lighter fluid on a pad of cotton, and place the pad over the tick for half a minute. Then pull the tick out.

(2) Coat each tick with Vaseline ® and then remove it with tweezers.

(3) Hold the lighted end of a cigarette very close to the tick, without actually touching it or the dog. The heat will make the tick withdraw its head, and it may then be removed.

If the head of the tick does break off: Clean the skin around the area with pHisoDerm ® or soap and water. Using a boiled (sterile) needle, remove the head of the tick from under your pet's skin exactly as you would remove a splinter from your own finger.

In tick-infested areas: Bathe the dog in a solution of .06% gamma benzene hexachloride (available at drugstores) every three weeks. This solution keeps the animal free of ticks.

Warts

Warts are small, round, pinkish lumps on the dog's skin, most frequently found around the muzzle and the top of the head.

The cause is not definitely known. Warts may be caused by a virus, or they may come from kissing frogs. In any case they are not serious, and since they will not trouble your dog, do not let them trouble you.

Treatment: Warts, which have a definite neck, may be removed by dog owners. Tie the wart off with a piece of cotton thread. In two or three days, the wart will drop off. Otherwise, warts are easily removed by a veterinarian.

ALLERGIES OF THE SKIN

Allergic Dermatitis

This condition is very common in dogs, especially during late summer.

Causes: An allergy to certain foods, varying from dog to dog. Hypersensitivity to fleas as well as synthetic carpet fibers can also be a cause.

Symptoms: The most obvious sign is intense itching and scratching which causes sore, weeping, red patches that often appear along the spine. If left untreated, the condition will not improve on its own.

Treatment: The object of treatment is to break the itch-scratch cycle. Shampoo the dog twice a week with a selenium sulfide shampoo (e.g., Seleen ®). Liberal amounts of soothing lotion, such as calamine lotion, should be applied to the affected areas twice a day. If the allergic dermatitis is caused by fleas, get rid of them. Try to help the dog break the itch-scratch cycle by bandaging its paws, or by tying baby booties on them. Even if the dog chews them off, it will provide a temporary respite from scratching.

Eczema

This common condition is a superficial inflammation of the skin and occurs in two forms: acute and chronic.

Acute:

Cause: Probably a severe allergic reaction.

Symptoms: Severe itching. The hairs around the affected areas are broken and sparse. The skin around the affected areas is bright red, moist and oozing. (In the long-haired breeds this may lead to the disease's going undetected, due to the matting of the animal's coat.)

Acute moist:

Symptoms: Constant scratching. This condition is typified by the sudden appearance of a large wet area exuding serum. (Serum is a yellowish fluid which dries to a yellowish crust.) Very painful breaks in the skin can appear overnight. These lesions are most common in areas that the animal can scratch or lick, and they vary in size from a penny to a hand. Initially, the breaks in the skin are wet and matted. Then they dry to a yellow scab. The pain is acute and obvious. The dog loses its appetite and is distressed.

Treatment: Apply a solution of 1:1,000 potassium permanganate crystals to the area (a pinch of crystals to 1 pint water—available at drugstores. Wash the entire dog with a shampoo containing selenium sulfide. After drying the animal, dab calamine lotion on the affected areas.

Chronic:

Causes: Dietary: excess carbohydrates; fat deficiency; vitamin deficiency; allergies; dirty skin; abrasions from collars or harnesses; friction between elbow and chest; overwashing; hormonal imbalance; individual predisposition; breed susceptibility (e.g., as in Scotties and Jack Russels).

In spayed females there may be scalding of the area around the vulva by urine. This occurs because bitches spayed before their first heat often retain an infantile vulva which remains small instead of developing to adult size.

Symptoms: The affected area becomes dry and flaky. The affected skin is darker than the rest of the skin.

Treatment: Seek professional help.

Labial eczema: A form of eczema which attacks the lips and is particularly common in spaniels.

Symptoms: The lips become raw and red, with the surrounding hair on the muzzle becoming brown-stained and foul-smelling.

Treatment: Clip away hair around the lips. Wash the area well with soap and water daily. Any good quality soap will do. For very severe cases: paint the sore areas with a silver nitrate stick (available from drugstores). Wear rubber gloves or you will burn your fingers. If home treatment is not successful, surgery may be necessary to remove the folds around the lips.

Nettle Rash and Hives (Urticaria)

Causes: Poison ivy; poison oak; stinging nettles; insect bites or stings; chemicals.

Symptoms: This is a common allergic reaction in dogs. The effect is very sudden: the eyelids and face may become swollen; round, clearly defined, raised patches will appear on the dog's body.

Treatment: If the animal is not in great discomfort, treatment may not be necessary. Most cases of nettle rash and hives clear up in six to eight hours. If the condition does not clear up, the vet will administer antihistamines and corticosteroids. This should give the animal quick relief.

If the hives are caused by an internal allergy, you won't be able to treat it at home, unless you know what the dog is allergic to. (See Allergies.) However, if it is caused by stinging nettles, and if the condition persists after twenty-four hours and professional help is not available, obtain an antihistamime cream (available at drugstores) and apply it to the affected area. Also administer diphenhydramine hydrochloride tablets. Dosage: 1 mg. per 3 pounds body weight. For puppies and elderly dogs, give 0.5 mg. per pound body weight.

INJURIES TO THE SKIN

Bee and Wasp Stings

Treatment: If you have seen the insect sting your dog, try to locate the stinger (it may be at the top of the swelling), and remove it by pinching at the bottom of the swelling with a pair of tweezers or a couple of wooden match sticks. (Only bees leave their stinger behind.) Do not try to pull out the stinger with your fingers. You will only succeed in squeezing the balance of the stinger's contents into your dog.

Bee stings: Bicarbonate of soda should be applied directly to the sting to relieve the pain.

Wasp stings: Apply vinegar directly over the sting. For stings on the mouth, use an ice pack to reduce the swelling.

Mild cases: Fortunately, most stings are not so severe and the pain usually subsides after half an hour.

For mild discomfort, lasting longer than half an hour, administer one-half of a 5-grain aspirin tablet per 20 pounds of body weight. (See How to Administer Tablets and Pills.)

If the swelling (or swellings) becomes very large (golf-ball size or larger), or if the dog has difficulty in breathing, get the animal to a vet immediately. If a vet is not available, try an animal-loving doctor, a dentist, or even a pharmacist. An injection of antihistamine is necessary.

Bruises and Contusions

Bruises and contusions are easy to see on the hairless parts of the animal, where the bruise is bluish red and painful to the touch.

If the bruise is under the hair, you will not be able to see it, but you can feel it and judge how severe it is by your dog's reaction.

Treatment: Examine the area around the bruise for breaks in the skin; these cuts and abrasions are often seen in association with bruises. If you find any cuts, clean and dress them. (See Cuts.) Apply hot compresses over the bruise for fifteen minutes, every two hours. If the dog is suffering marked discomfort, administer an analgesic.

Burns and Scalds

Burns and scalds are the most common household accidents, and the dog owner should familiarize himself with the treatment of these mishaps *before* they happen.

A burn is caused by dry heat, such as a flame. A scald is caused by moist heat, such as steam. But the difference is academic, since symptoms and treatment are the same for both conditions.

Treatment: When handling or treating a dog that has been burned, be careful. Burns are very painful and animals in pain resent being handled. A good tape muzzle or a competent assistant is essential. (See Restraint and Handling.)

In serious cases, where the dog has been badly burned, treat first for shock. Keep the dog warm and give it a mixture of glucose and water. Relieve the pain by administering an analgesic: one 5-grain aspirin tablet for small dogs, up to 25 grains for large dogs, once only. (See How to Administer Tablets and Pills.) Then clean the area around the burn with a dilute solution of pHisoDerm ® (1 teaspoon to 1 pint water) to remove any damaged tissue (burned or charred skin). Apply tannic acid jelly (available at drugstores) or a solution of cooled strong tea to the burned area. Bandage the area to prevent further fluid loss, which can lead to serious problems. In very severe cases, wrap the dog up in a blanket and get it to a vet.

Long-haired dogs: It usually takes two or three days before any signs appear. Then a sticky green crust forms on the skin. Do not pull this crust off. It will come off naturally leaving a large, pinkish weeping area. If it does not come away, bathe it or soak it off. Then clean the area and use a little cod-liver oil on a cotton pad for the dressing.

In very severe cases with associated shock, a vet will give stimulants and plasma to combat fluid loss. (See Shock: Transportation of Injured Dogs.)

Chemical Burns

Causes: Caustic soda, sulfuric acid, hydrochloric acid, diesel oil, etc. (Animals often come into contact with diesel oil when they go under a parked truck.)

Symptoms: A chemical burn resembles a scald. The wound is moist and oozing. The hair around the burn usually sloughs off. If the dog has tried to drink the chemical, there will be ulcers around its muzzle and tongue.

Treatment: Use soap and water to wash the chemical off the dog's hair and skin. For acid burns, apply dilute bicarbonate of soda to the burned area. For alkali burns apply vinegar and water. If you do not know whether the burn was caused by an acid or an alkali, simply wash the affected area with soap and water. Apply dilute pHisoHex ® to the burn. Apply tannic acid jelly (available at drugstores) or a solution of cooled, strong tea to the burned area. Bandage the area to prevent further fluid loss. It is this loss of fluid that creates serious problems in burn cases. In very severe cases, wrap the dog in a blanket and get it to a vet.

Long-haired dogs: If a long-haired dog is burned, it usually takes two or three days before any signs appear. Then a sticky green crust forms on the skin. Do not pull this crust off. It will come off by itself, leaving a large pinkish, weeping area. If it does not come off, bathe it off or soak it off. Then clean and dress the area, using a little cod-liver oil on a gauze pad for the dressing.

In very severe cases with associated shock, a vet will give stimulants and plasma to combat fluid loss. (See Shock; Transportation of Injured Dogs.)

Cuts

Treatment: For simple cuts: wash the wound with a saline solution, then examine it to be sure that all foreign matter, such as grit, sand, etc., has been removed. (See Saline Solution.)

If foreign objects are visible, but embedded too deeply

to come out easily, apply a kaolin poultice. (See Poultices.) After the wound has been cleansed, disinfect and dress it with a 10% solution of hydrogen peroxide. Do not bandage the cut unless the dog bothers it.

Frostbite

In this condition, destruction of tissue is caused by exposure to severe cold. The parts of the body most often frostbitten are the nose, toes, tips of the ears, and tip of the tail.

Mild cases: Frostbitten skin becomes cold and white; loss of hair around the affected parts.

Severe cases: Loss of hair, followed by redness and localized pain.

In even more serious cases, the area remains sore, sensitive to touch, swells, then shrivels. Finally, the skin around the affected area sloughs away, leaving an open weeping surface.

Treatment: In mild cases, increase the circulation of the blood to the frostbitten area by rubbing the area briskly with your hand. Then apply camphor oil or oil of wintergreen. If the dog is very uncomfortable, an aspirin (from 5 to 25 grains, depending upon size, may be administered once only in a twenty-four-hour period. (See How to Administer Tablets and Pills.)

Seek professional help. In extreme cases, amputation may be necessary. (See Gangrene.)

Jellyfish Stings

Symptoms: These vary according to the species of jellyfish and the site of the sting. Generally speaking, if the dog exhibits certain extreme symptoms and obvious pain after swimming in the sea, treat for jellyfish sting.

Treatment: Relieve the pain. Begin by making certain that there are no tentacles of the jellyfish clinging to the dog's skin. (Be careful when removing tentacles; they can still sting!) If the dog is suffering more than mild discomfort, administer one-half tablet to two tablets of aspirin, depending upon body weight. Local applications of olive oil or bicarbonate of soda are also helpful. If available, a solution of dilute ammonia (1 part ammonia to 10 parts of water) applied at once will prevent most of the painful results of the sting.

Severe cases: In severe cases, the symptoms will be much more serious. The dog owner will not have the necessary medicines for alleviating the toxic effects of the sting. So, in these extreme cases, he can only treat any symptoms of shock that may appear. (See Shock.)

Keep the dog warm. Give it a solution of 4 tablespoons of glucose added to 1 pint of water. For small dogs give 4 ounces of this solution, up to 1 pint for large dogs. In severe cases, the dog may stop breathing; be prepared to administer artificial respiration. (See Artificial Respiration.)

In these extreme cases, get the dog to a vet.

Leash Clips Caught in the Flesh

Occasionally, when a leash clip is being attached to a dog's collar, the clip becomes attached to the loose folds of the dog's neck. It may also become attached to the web between the toes.

Treatment: If the clip is deeply embedded in the skin, do not try to take it off the way you got it on. First apply a tape muzzle. (See Restraint and Handling.) Then cut off the back of the clip with a hacksaw or wire cutters. If you do not have the tools, try the nearest garage.

Prevention: Do not use leash clips that are shaped like a question mark; get the type with jointed action.

Poison on the Skin

If a poison has contacted the skin or hair, bathe the affected parts with soap and water. Even if the poison does not burn the skin, it must be removed immediately, otherwise the dog will lick its coat and ingest the poison. (See Poisoning.)

Porcupines

Technique for removing porcupine quills: Use tweezers or pliers and remove the quills, one at a time, by twisting each quill one full turn clockwise. Then pull—do not jerk—the quill out.

Skunks

Technique for neutralizing skunk spray: Wash the entire dog in tomato juice, taking care not to get it in the dog's eyes. This will have the effect of removing the skunk smell.

Skunk spray in the eyes: Wash the dog's eyes out with clean, cool water. Badly inflamed eyes call for a vet's skill.

Snake Bite

Treatment: Dogs are usually bitten on the legs, so apply two tourniquets, one above and one below the bite.

The quickest way to make a tourniquet is to take a handkerchief or tear a strip of material, wrap it around the limb, insert a pencil or stick into the tourniquet on the side of the wound nearest the heart, then twist. Be sure to loosen the tourniquet every twenty minutes. Then retighten it.

The purpose of the tourniquet is to prevent the poison from passing from the site of the bite into the bloodstream. To this end, ice packs and cold dressings, when available, should also be applied to the site.

The fang marks, when visible, should be enlarged by making two simple incisions, one on either side of the bite, with a razor blade or penknife. Then the venom should be sucked out.

Then apply potassium permanganate crystals (available at drugstores) to the site of the bite. When traveling through snake country, it would be wise to carry a small supply.

If the dog has been bitten by a seriously venomous snake, the only effective treatment is an intravenous injection of antivenin.

Keep the dog as quiet as possible. The faster its heart beats, the faster the venom is distributed through its system. Seek professional help.

Warning: Antihistamines should not be administered.

Wounds

A wound is a break or lesion of the body surfaces. When the wound occurs, the dog bleeds. Usually, if the wound is superficial and the bleeding slight, the blood will clot and the bleeding will stop. But if the dog is losing a lot of blood, first aid must be administered.

Treatment: The first priority is to stop the bleeding, regardless of whether it is arterial or venous. If the dog is bleeding very badly, do not waste time. Jam a wad of rags, Kleenex ®, or a towel over the wound. Press hard and hold it there until the bleeding stops. If nothing else is available, use your hand or fingers pressed directly on the wound to stop the bleeding.

Once you have stanched the wound, try to determine whether it is arterial or venous. If the blood is bright red and spurting, it comes from a severed artery. If the blood is deeper red and oozing, it comes from a vein. For arterial wounds, apply a tourniquet between the wound and the heart. For venous wounds, the tourniquet is applied on the side of the wound farthest from the heart.

If the wound is on the trunk or the neck, where a tourniquet cannot be used, keep pressing the wad of material or your hand over the wound until the bleeding stops. When you do remove the pressure, be careful not to tear away the protective clotting and start the wound bleeding again.

Once the bleeding has been controlled, the next step depends upon the severity of the injury and whether or not the dog is in a state of shock. If it is, then it must be treated for shock. If not, proceed to treat the wound. (See Shock, under Transportation of Injured Dogs.)

Dressing the wound: Clip the hair around the wound with blunt-pointed scissors. Wash the wound with soap (any good-quality hand soap) and cooled, boiled water. If you have an antiseptic (e.g., pHisoDerm ®) handy, use it. Otherwise, soap and water will do. Be sure to wash away the dirt, oil, or grease from the center of the wound. After drying, apply a simple dressing to keep out infection. A pad of cotton secured with adhesive tape will do the job. Change the dressing once a day. For severe wounds, after cleaning and dressing, contact a vet.

The most efficacious treatment for a wound can be determined by observing the kind of wound it is.

Classification of wounds:

(1) Clean *incised wounds* bleed freely, and a pressure bandage or tourniquet should be applied.

(2) *Lacerated wounds* are jagged, irregular wounds that bleed minimally and require ordinary bandaging.

(3) *Puncture wounds* are usually the result of bites and are nearly always infected.

(4) When accompanied by bruising, they are known as *contused wounds.*

THE HAIR

Baldness (Alopecia)

Causes: This condition is common in dogs and may occur without any visible cause. Baldness may be the result of an iodine deficiency, a hormonal imbalance, or certain generalized illnesses.

Symptoms: The hair falls out in patches, which may or may not itch.

Treatment: Apply an iodine and glycerine solution (1 part of 2% tincture of iodine mixed with 30 parts of glycerin) directly to the bald patches. The vet may administer an oral dose of thyroid hormone: 30 mg. per 10 pounds body weight. Oral administration of corticosteroids will also help to relieve the itching, but must be prescribed by a vet.

Dandruff (Scurf)

This condition is common in dogs with dry coats. Dog dandruff looks exactly like human dandruff: fine white flakes scattered throughout the coat, especially along the spine.

Treatment: This condition should be promptly treated to prevent it from becoming a problem.

Shampoo the dog every three days for two weeks with a selenium sulfide shampoo (e.g., Seleen ®).

In addition to the shampoo, give a small dog 1 tablespoon of corn oil daily for a week; feed larger dogs 2 tablespoons daily for a week.

Dogs with a tendency toward dandruff should have regular amounts of corn oil added to their diets: 4-6 tablespoons a week (depending on size) should prevent the condition from recurring.

Paint Removal

Technique: Get some dry cloths and rub off all the paint you can. Wash small areas thoroughly with soap and water and keep rubbing with cloths. Snip off patches of matted hair with scissors. For particularly difficult patches, pour a little rubbing alcohol on the patch and then rub off with a dry cloth. Hand cleaners, such as Boraxo ®, may also be used.

Warning: Never use kerosene, turpentine, or any of the paint solvents. They cause burns on the dog's skin.

Lead in paints: Paints which contain led are poisonous when ingested. If a dog has eaten paint with a lead base, or has licked paint off its coat, force-feed 1 bowl of milk with 2 egg whites beaten into it. (See Force Feeding.) If lead poisoning is suspected, do not try to induce vomiting.

If the dog is in pain, or is covered with paint, get it to a vet. Often a general anesthetic is necessary and, in severe cases, intravenous fluids must be administered to combat shock. Even lead-free paints can be a powerful irritant. Also, many paints contain poisonous coal tar derivatives.

Shedding (Loss of Hair)

A certain degree of shedding is natural, occurring twice a year, during the spring and autumn. If the dog loses large amounts of hair at other times, make sure that the animal is being properly groomed. If regular grooming has been carried out, this loss of hair should be considered abnormal.

Causes: Shedding may be due to thyroid deficiency; chronic nephritis; malnutrition; hormone deficiency; or fatty acid deficiency.

General treatment: Bathe and groom the dog, using a selenium sulfide shampoo. Adding corn oil to the shedding dog's diet (1 teaspoon a week for a small dog, up to 5 tablespoons a week for a large dog) should improve the condition.

4

Problems of
the Chest

ALLERGIES OF THE RESPIRATORY TRACT

Allergic Asthma

This is not a common condition, but when it does occur it must be treated or it can develop into something even more serious.

Symptoms: Usually occurs in summer months. Affected dogs become short-winded and wheezy.

Treatment: Administer tablets of Benadryl ® (diphenhydramine hydrochloride). Dosage: 1 mg. per pound body weight twice a day. For elderly dogs, give 0.5 mg. per pound body weight. (See How to Administer Tablets and Pills.)

Hay Fever

Hay fever, an allergy of the nose and throat (upper respiratory tract) sometimes occurs in dogs.

Symptoms: Sneezing, accompanied by running eyes and nose, during period of high pollen count (dates vary with locale).

Treatment: Administer Benadryl ® (diphenhydramine hydrochloride tablets). Dosage: 1 mg. per pound of body weight up to three times a day. For elderly dogs and puppies, give 0.5 mg. per pound body weight. (See How to Administer Tablets and Pills.)

BRONCHITIS, EXCESSIVE COUGHING AND KENNEL COUGH

Bronchitis, Excessive Coughing:
Symptoms: Excessive coughing, often with phlegm.
Treatment: First, get a good light and examine the dog's throat to make sure that the cough is not caused by a foreign body in the mouth or throat. Then, treat the cough with cough syrup, 1 teaspoon per 20 pounds body weight, three times a day. Diet: no food for twenty-four hours. Then a light diet of fish or chicken. If, after forty-eight hours, your dog is still coughing excessively, find a vet.

Kennel Cough:
Symptoms: A dry cough, unaccompanied by phlegm.
Causes: It is caused by a viruslike organism, which responds poorly to antibiotics.
Treatment: Administer codeine tablets: 8 mg. per pound of body weight, to a maximum of 40 mg. per day, until the condition improves. If untreated, the dog usually coughs for five or six weeks before the condition recedes. But though the cough goes, if the condition is not treated the dog may be left with impaired breathing. So when coughing persists, see a vet. If professional help is not available, home treatment is an obligation.

CHEST WOUNDS

Treatment: Place a moistened gauze pad or wad of material directly over the wound.

Place a plastic bag or sheet over the pad and secure it with adhesive or Scotch ® tape, to obtain an airtight shield over the wound.

In an emergency, do not waste time looking for a pad or wad of material. Use your hand or fingers to stop the bleeding. Put your hand or fingers directly on the bleeding wound, and press. This should stop the bleeding until you can dress the wound properly.

If the wound continues to bleed through the dressing, apply another pad and bandage it tighter, or apply more pressure by hand over the wound. Do not remove the first dressing. This will disturb the blood clot which is forming over the wound and increase the bleeding.

Transporting a dog with a chest wound: Move a wounded dog only when you must. If you can hear air sucking in and out of the wound, carry the dog with its breastbone down. Otherwise, carry the animal with the wound uppermost.

COLDS

Dogs do not catch colds. But if a dog shows symptoms of the common cold, do not treat these symptoms lightly. The symptoms (runny nose, coughing, shivering, etc.) suggest something more serious. (See Distemper Complex; Sinusitis; Nosebleed.)

Pleurisy

Pleurisy is an inflammation of the pleura, the membrane that surrounds the lungs and lines the walls of the chest.

Symptoms: Pleurisy produces the same symptoms as pneumonia: a high fever, painful and difficult breathing, loss of appetite, and lethargy.

Treatment: Pleurisy, like pneumonia, cannot be accurately diagnosed or adequately treated by a nonprofessional. Home treatment consists of keeping the dog warm and trying to get it to take some nourishment and to drink plenty of fluids.

It must be stressed that pleurisy should be considered a serious illness, and suspicion of pleurisy warrants an immediate consultation with a vet.

Pneumonia

Pneumonia is an infection of the lungs.

Causes: Viruses; bacteria; worms. Sometimes a simple chill, if left untreated, can develop into penumonia.

Symptoms: General symptoms include coughing, lethargy, dullness, high fever. Also check the dog for bluish-tinged mucous membranes. There is a rattling and bubbling in the dog's chest. Often the afflicted dog will lie on its breastbone, with its elbow stuck out at a 45° angle. This is caused by the sore chest that accompanies pneumonia. When the dog is picked up, there is further evidence of pain in its chest, because its lungs are sore and picking it up compresses the lungs and increases the soreness.

Treatment: Pneumonia is a serious disease and professional aid should be sought. If a vet is not immediately available, the owner must make certain that the dog is kept warm. Wrap it in a blanket or a woolen sweater, or button a cardigan around it. Also, be sure that the room where the dog is kept is warm, and at the same time make sure there is adequate fresh air. Try to tempt the dog's appetite with light, nourishing food. Give plenty of fluids.

5

Problems of the Abdomen

THE STOMACH

Flatulence (Breaking Wind)

This condition often occurs in dogs that are: overweight, underexercised, suffering from a dietary imbalance; suffering from a bowel infection.

Treatment: If your older dog is eating one large meal a day, start feeding it two or three smaller meals per day. Check to be sure that you are not overfeeding. (See Diet.) Remove liver, heart, and milk from the diet. Allow the dog more opportunity to exercise. If reducing the size of meals and increasing exercise does not help, add a handful of charcoal to the dog's food each day.

Emergency: Occasionally, a dog will break wind excessively and will suddenly become quite bloated. Its abdomen becomes swollen with gas and hard. This is an emergency.

Death may result from torsion (twisted stomach). Do not poke or probe the distended abdomen.

There is no effective first aid for this acute condition. Get the dog to a vet immediately.

Hiccups

Causes: Puppies that bolt their food often get hiccups. They also get hiccups if their stomachs are empty. Occasionally, the adult dog will also develop hiccups.

Adult dogs: The condition is not serious and usually disappears naturally. However, if the hiccups persist for more than half an hour, administer 1 tablespoon milk of magnesia. (See Force Feeding.)

Puppies: There is no need to worry about hiccups in puppies. If the pup appears distressed, put a little olive oil on your finger and rub the pup's abdomen to induce burping.

ABDOMINAL DISORDERS

Swelling of the Abdomen

Symptoms: A sudden and dramatic increase in the size of the abdomen suggests: overeating; pregnancy; tumors; fluid in the abdomen as a result of liver or heart failure; pyometra; ovarian cyst; enlargement of the liver; enlargement of the spleen; torsion of the stomach.

Treatment: If the symptoms described under these entries (see Index) are similar to those exhibited by your dog, consult a veterinarian. Although the first signs of these conditions may not constitute an emergency, your alertness can help to prevent the serious complications that may develop.

Gastroenteritis

Gastroenteritis is a general term for an infection of the stomach and intestines which is characterized by vomiting and diarrhea.

Fever stage: High fever; loss of appetite; lethargy; depression; possible abdominal pain.

A dog with a high fever will have dull eyes, a worn expression, a dry, hot nose, and a dry coat. Dogs with abdominal pain often lie with their rear legs up and their front legs extended. They tend to seek out cold places, such as cement floors, to lie on, and they are restless.

Vomiting stage: Continual vomiting. Initially, the vomit is white and frothy, then it becomes yellow. In advanced stages, it may be bloodstained. During the vomiting stage, the dog will be very thirsty. It will drink and then vomit, setting in motion the drink-vomit cycle.

Diarrhea stage: Once the vomiting stage has been established, diarrhea usually begins. About twenty-four hours later, it becomes bloodstained.

Treatment: Withhold food and water for twenty-four hours. Consult a vet.

Heartworms

Although this disease mainly affects dogs living along the eastern seaboard, and in some Gulf States, instances of heartworm have been reported on the West Coast as well.

Cause: Heartworms are parasites which are carried and transmitted by mosquitoes.

The conditon occurs in two forms: a common chronic form, and a rarer, acute hepatic form, which attacks the liver and kidneys.

Chronic Form: The first symptom is a constant dry cough, which becomes worse when the dog is exercising. This coughing is coupled with shortness of breath, caused by the formation of fluid in the chest and abdomen. Other symptoms include red-stained urine and palpitations of the heart.

Acute form: There are no initial signs such as coughing or shortness of breath. In this form, death can occur within twenty-four to seventy-two hours after the main symptom, which is blood in the urine. Death is due to combined liver and kidney failure.

Treatment: There is no home treatment for this disease. Dog owners living in heartworm areas should get professional advice before the condition appears. Prevention is the key. There are pills that can be fed to a dog during the mosquito season (dates vary with locale) to prevent the growth of these worms.

Hernia

A hernia is the protrusion of internal tissue through a natural opening which would normally close in the course of growth (e.g., the navel or the inguinal canal in the groin). There are four types of hernia: umbilical, inguinal, scrotal, and traumatic. However, the traumatic is not a true hernia.

Umbilical hernia: Seen fairly frequently in puppies.

Symptoms: There is a small protrusion of intestinal fat visible at the navel.

Treatment: This form of hernia is not often serious if the bit of fat protruding is pliable and small, a quarter of an inch or less. The puppy grows, but the protrusion remains small. So leave it alone.

If the protruding portion is larger, the pup should be taken to a vet for minor surgery.

Inguinal hernia: A swelling in the groin which continues to grow. Most bitches have tiny inguinal hernias.

Treatment: While many small hernias do not require treatment, it is best to seek professional advice. Surgical intervention may be needed.

Scrotal hernia: A swelling of the scrotum.

Symptoms: This swelling is particularly noticeable after the dog has eaten a heavy meal. There may be discomfort and, in severe cases, acute pain and possible strangulation of the bowel.

Treatment: Surgical.

Emergency: If the pain is obviously acute, seek professional assistance without delay. The danger comes from possible strangulation of the bowel, and this constitutes an emergency.

Traumatic hernia: This occurs after accidents and requires immediate professional treatment.

Internal Hemorrhage

Causes: Road accidents, falls, and eating anticoagulant poisons (warfarin, mouse and rat poison) can produce internal bleeding.

Symptoms: The overall symptoms are the same as those in cases of severe shock: pronounced weakness and heavy panting; fast, weak pulse rate; pale mucous membranes around the lips and nose; cold paws.

Treatment: There is no first aid treatment for this condition. The only certain way of controlling the bleeding is surgical.

Emergency: If these symptoms are observed, do not waste time. Wrap the dog in a blanket and get it to a vet.

Have someone telephone the vet first, if possible, so that he can have the necessary preparations ready when you arrive.

Intestinal Protrusion

Dogs involved in fights or a variety of accidents (e.g., road accidents, jumping on fences) may tear their abdominal wall to such an extent that the internal organs protrude.

This is a serious emergency, but it need not be fatal. The real danger lies in the possibility of internal hemorrhage, shock, or accidental self-mutilation. Immediate first aid can prevent these complications.

Treatment: Assess the damage: if there is no vet available, be prepared to do more than just bandage the wound. Calm the dog. Try not to touch the wound more than you have to. If the protruding portions of the intestines are dirty, they should be washed gently in boiled water which has been cooled. Pour the water over the protruding part of the intestines. If only a small portion of the intestine protrudes, gently push it back into the dog's abdomen through the wound. Place a sterile gauze pad over the wound and bandage the pad around the dog's body. Treat for shock if necessary. (See Shock.) Seek professional help immediately.

6

Problems of the Anorectal Region

ABNORMAL STOOLS

An abnormal bowel movement is distinguished from a normal one by: (1) *Texture:* Hard (constipation); soft (diarrhea). (2) *Color:* Blood in feces (consult a vet; it could be an ulcer or a tumor); too pale (suspect gall bladder or pancreas problems); too dark (there could be blood in the stool). (3) *Quantity:* More than usual; less than usual; flat, ribbonlike movement. (4) *Unusual objects in feces:* Worms, bits of bone, etc. (5) *Odor:* Foul, oily, rancid smell.

The signs of abnormal bowel movements usually appear in conjunction with other symptoms. If the signs listed above are observed, seek professional advice without delay.

Blood in Stools

A small amount of blood in the feces is seen from time to

time in all meat-eating animals. Larger amounts of blood are not normal and should not be ignored.

Causes: Blood in the feces may be the result of anal impaction, such as bones, or may be caused by tumors of the rectum, canine hepatitis, poisoning, or accidents.

Symptoms: Bright red, fresh blood coming from the anal region; black blood coming from the intestines.

Treatment: Unless the cause can be easily identified and treated (e.g., bones or a simple cut), have a vet examine the dog. Home treatment is empirical, that is, treat the symptoms. Give no food until the bleeding stops.

Constipation

Causes: Often occurs in dogs which are fed bones; in male dogs with enlarged prostate glands; rectal tumors; abdominal tumors; loss of muscle tone in muscles surrounding the anus (as a result of improper tail docking); anal gland abscesses; slipped disks; and after badly treated, healed pelvic fractures.

Symptoms: Straining; passing a brown, watery discharge; bleeding from the anus; vomiting.

Treatment: Administer 3–5 tablespoons (depending on size) of mineral oil and starve the dog.

If the dog has not had a bowel movement within twenty-four hours after receiving the laxative, contact a vet. The cause of the constipation may be more serious and an enema may be necessary.

Diarrhea

Diarrhea is the name of a condition in which loose, unformed feces are passed.

Causes: Dogs are natural scavengers and often suffer mild attacks of diarrhea as a result of eating decayed food. However, it can also be caused by viruses, bacteria, intestinal parasites, or poisons.

Symptoms: Frequent passage of loose stool; foul-smelling feces; sometimes associated with vomiting.

Treatment: All food and water should be withheld for twenty-four hours. After twenty-four hours, feed a cup of water a day and small amounts of deboned chicken and rice or fish and rice for the next two or three days. *No milk should be given for one week.*

If the diarrhea persists, starve the dog for another twenty-four hours. Then feed the following mixture: mix 3–4 tablespoons glucose, 1 raw egg white, 1 pinch salt into 1 pint warm water. Give the dog 2 tablespoons of this mixture every two hours for two days. (See Force Feeding.) Put the animal on a reduced diet of deboned chicken and rice or fish and rice for the next two or three days. Then resume normal feeding.

Severe diarrhea may also be controlled by administering Enterovioform tablets (Ciba): one tablet per 20 pounds body weight three times a day for no longer than two days. (See How to Administer Tablets and Pills.)

Persistent diarrhea: If diarrhea persists for more than forty-eight hours, it may be the symptom of a more serious disease such as distemper or leptospirosis. A vet must be consulted.

Sore anus: Dogs with diarrhea may develop a sore anus. Apply Vaseline ® or cold cream to the anal area every two hours.

Prolapse of the Rectum

This condition is fairly common in puppies suffering from persistent diarrhea. Occasionally, it is also seen in older dogs.

Treatment: Wash your hands, then gently wash the area around the anus with warm, soapy water. Apply mineral oil liberally around the anal area. Gently push back the protruding portion until the anus is normal.

ANAL GLANDS

The anal glands, the size of a hazelnut, are circular glands located inside the anus at the four o'clock and eight o'clock positions. When the anal gland does not empty itself normally and becomes overfull, it must be emptied by manipulation.

Symptoms: The dog smells of feces and continually rubs its bottom on the ground.

Technique for emptying glands: Hold the tail in your left hand. With the right hand, make a ring of your index finger and thumb. Squeeze the ring with a slow but firm action against the base of the anus. Discharge comes as the glands are emptied.

The anal gland should not be emptied more than once every two months, or permanent damage may occur.

Anal eczema: When acute eczemas in this area are being treated, the anal gland should be suspected of causing the eczema and, as a part of the treatment, the anal gland should be emptied.

Emptying the anal gland is not difficult, but it would be helpful if the dog owner were to watch a vet do it once.

Anal Gland Abscesses

Symptoms: Very painful red swellings under the anus, on one or both sides.

Treatment: Apply hot compresses to the area for ten minutes at a time, four times a day, until the swelling subsides. If the compresses are not effective after forty-eight hours, it may be necessary to lance the abscess. If a veterinarian is not available, the owner may lance the abscess himself.

Technique for lancing: Boil a single-edge razor blade for twenty minutes. Clean the skin around the abscess with a disinfecting solution of pHisoDerm ® and alcohol (1 teaspoon of each to 1 pint water). Have an assistant hold the dog's head tightly, or tie the dog's mouth shut. (See Restraint and Handling.) Make a half-inch incision over the softest, reddest point of the swelling. Allow the abscess to drain.

Anal Tumors (Adenoma)

Anal adenoma is a local malignant tumor seen only in older male dogs. It takes the form of one or more swellings around the anorectal area or on the tail. In advanced cases, these swellings may ulcerate and hemorrhage.

Treatment: Effective and lasting treatment must be by a professional. In advanced cases, surgery may be required; in less advanced cases, antibiotics and hormones will probably help.

While this condition is not an emergency, it must not be neglected. All too often a dog owner is not even aware that it exists until the dog begins bleeding, and what is originally a simple problem becomes a more serious one. If bleeding occurs, hold a pad over the bleeding area (bandaging this area would be very difficult) and get the dog to a vet.

WORMS

Worms: General (See also Ringworm, Heartworm)

Worms are one of several types of parasites that may try to use your dog as their host. Unpleasant as they are, worms rarely cause serious problems, except in puppies. During the first eight months of the dog's life, the owner should be alert to the possibility of worms.

Causes: The worms are picked up from other animals and from feces of affected animals.

Young dogs: Worms in young dogs produce a variety of symptoms that may be seen separately or in combination with each other: vomiting of worms; worms in the feces; potbelly; halitosis; stunted growth.

Adult dogs: In adult dogs, worms are rarely detected until they are either coughed up or appear in the feces.

Warning: While most types of worms are not particularly dangerous to the dog itself, the roundworm can be transmitted to humans and may cause blindness. This is one more good reason why children should not be encouraged to let stray puppies lick their faces, and a good reason for insisting that they wash their hands before eating, after playing with any animal, including their own.

Since the dog owner cannot make a definite diagnosis of hookworm, whipworm, roundworm, etc., it is advisable to treat all worms and suspected worm conditions with hygienic precaution.

Treatment: For worms other than tapeworms, administer piperazine tablets (available from drugstores), 500 mg. per 10 pounds of body weight. Repeat after one week.

Tapeworms

Symptoms: Tapeworms rarely cause any severe or dramatic symptoms, apart from a change in the texture and color of the coat. There may be some non-specific illness and diarrhea. By "non-specific" illness we mean that the dog may be off form; nothing specific, nothing you can put your finger on, just not well. The observant owner will notice segments of tapeworms in the feces, and other segments sticking to the fur around the anus.

Description: The dog owner will have no difficulty in distinguishing the tapeworms. When freshly passed, these segments are about one-quarter inch long, moist, and quite active. They dry rapidly and shrivel up. When dry, they resemble small, brownish grains of rice, and are often found in the dog's bedding.

Treatment: Fortunately, treatment is simple and usually effective. There are a number of excellent commercial tapeworm preparations available (e.g., Dicestal ®, or Teniathane ®). Administer 500 mg. per 6 pounds of body weight, after a meal. Wait seven days and repeat the dose. Since tapeworm eggs are carried by the flea, get rid of the fleas as well as the tapeworms. (See Fleas.)

7

Problems of the Urinary System

Bladder Infection (Cystitis)

An infection of the bladder, fairly common in dogs.

Symptoms: Blood or traces of blood in the urine; passing urine with increased frequency; straining to pass urine; loss of appetite; abdominal pain. In later stages, the urine will be heavily bloodstained. As the disease progresses, pure blood will be passed.

Treatment: Do not feed the dog until professional help is available. If it takes longer than twenty-four hours to get a vet, glucose and water may be given. (See Urethral Obstructions and Bladder Stones.)

Chronic Interstitial Nephritis (Kidney Failure)

This condition is frequently seen in elderly dogs (seven years or older) following an infection of leptospirosis. (See Leptospirosis.)

Symptoms: The dog is constantly thirsty and, as a result, begins to pass more urine than usual. Its physical condition deteriorates. The coat is dull and there are skin eruptions. As the condition progresses, the dog vomits frequently and suffers from diarrhea and excessive urination and thirst. The dog's breath is bad; the urine is pale and passed in larger quantities than normally.

The disease occurs in two forms: compensated and decompensated. In the compensated form, the dog drinks excessively and is able to flush the poison through its kidneys. In the decompensated form, the dog is unable to flush the accumulated poisons out of its body and may die.

Treatment: The dog must be given as much clean water as it can drink. Make sure that its water bowl is always full. Feed the dog a low-protein diet of the white meat from deboned chicken or fish, or a commercially prepared nephritis diet available from the vet and pet stores. Antibiotic treatment may be helpful, but this must be left to the discretion of the vet.

Discharge from the Penis (Balantis)

Cause: This condition is a result of an inflammation of the penis.

Symptoms: There is a continuing discharge or dripping of yellowish pus from the dog's sheath.

Treatment: Pull the penis out of its sheath and bathe the head and exposed shank in an antiseptic solution (e.g., pHisoDerm ®). Then use water to wash off the pHisoDerm ®. Do this three times a day until the inflammation and discharge disappear. If the animal will not allow you to pull out its penis, then syringe the inside of the sheath with a solution of 4 parts water to 1 part pHisoDerm ®. This syringing should be done three or four times a day until the condition disappears. It may sound like a difficult operation, but most dogs are surprisingly cooperative and do not seem to mind the bathing procedure.

Irretractable Penis (Paraphimosis)

In this condition the penis protrudes from the sheath instead of sliding back into place.

Causes: The sheath opening is too small; hypersexuality.

Treatment: Apply warm olive oil to the shaft of the penis. Then, gently manipulate it back into the sheath. With smaller dogs, simply plunge them into a cold bath. The penis should retract automatically.

Prostatitis (Enlarged Prostate Gland)

The prostate gland is found only in the male animal.

Causes: Old age; hypersexuality.

Symptoms: Straining and obvious pain when having a bowel movement. Passage of flattened or ribbon feces.

Treatment: Problems with the prostate gland are serious and require professional treatment. Antibiotics and, possibly, female hormones may be indicated.

If a vet is not immediately available, administer mineral oil (1–3 tablespoons, depending on size of dog) to enable the dog to pass a bowel movement with less difficulty. (See Constipation.)

Urethral Obstructions and Bladder Stones (Cystic Calculi)

The urethra is the tube through which urine is passed from the bladder to the outside of the body. Occasionally this tube becomes irritated or, in severe cases, blocked.

Cause: Depending upon the seriousness of the symptoms, this condition could be caused by a mild cystitis infection, bladder stones, or complete blockage of the urethra. Blockage of the urethra is serious and must be treated without delay.

Symptoms: Inability to pass urine; distended abdomen; standing in a peculiar, splay-legged position; profound depression and apathy.

Emergency: If your dog displays these symptoms, this is an emergency. You must get professional help immediately. Do not attempt to prod the distended abdomen or the bladder may rupture. If this happens, the dog will die.

8

Problems of
the Extremities

Amputation

Amputation is the removal of one or more limbs either surgically or traumatically.

Surgical amputation: Severe fractures, bone cancers, or very severe cases of arthritis sometimes make amputation necessary. Many dog owners are naturally reluctant to allow this operation, even though the animal's life is at stake. Some owners would rather have their pets "put away" than have them hobbling about on three legs. If this reluctance is analyzed, it usually turns out that the objection is basically due to the cosmetic effect of amputation. Owners faced with this decision should know that dogs learn fairly rapidly to compensate for a missing limb and are able to manage quite well on three legs. As for appearances, it is amazing how quickly even the most sensitive dog owners become accustomed to their pets' lack of appendages.

Traumatic amputation: This occurs during accidents. A

138

tourniquet must be applied immediately. Measures must be taken to prevent or minimize the effects of shock, while the dog is being transported to the vet. (See Shock; Tourniquet.)

If possible, have someone telephone the vet so that he can have the necessary transfusions ready when the animal arrives. Don't worry about saving a severed limb to be sewn on later (unless, of course, you happen to have Dr. Barnard for your vet).

Cracked Pads

Symptoms: If a dog is suffering from a cracked pad, it will be lame on hard surfaces but sound when walking on grass. Before you decide that your dog has a cracked pad, examine the paw carefully in a good light to be sure that it is not a cut pad. (See Wounds.) (Cut pads are much more common, especially in city dogs.)

Also check to be sure that the lameness is not caused by a cracked nail, particularly a dewclaw.

Treatment: Treat a cracked or sore pad by bathing the paw in a solution made by adding 10 tea bags to 1 pint of boiling water. Allow the tea to cool and add 4 tablespoons of witch hazel. Continue the bathing twice a day for one week.

Rub a little olive oil into the pad. Then tie a baby bootie around the paw for a few days. If the dog chews the bootie off, bandage the paw with an adhesive bandage. (See Bandaging the Leg.) If the dog bites at the bandage, use an Elizabethan collar. (See Elizabethan Collar.) It is also helpful to walk the dog on grass rather than on hard surfaces, until the pad heals.

In general, if a cut or cracked pad is not bleeding, the less treatment the better. After the cracked pad has healed, encourage the animal to walk. This will make the pad harden sooner.

Dewclaws

The dewclaw is a functionless toe that appears as a rudimentary claw on the lower, inside part of the dog's leg just above the paw.

Since dewclaws serve no purpose, and may catch on material, it is recommended that they be removed not earlier than three days, nor later than ten days after birth. After ten days, professional assistance is required.

Technique for removing dewclaws in puppies: Sterilize a sharp pair of scissors by boiling them in water for twenty minutes. Clean the skin around the dewclaws with a solution of dilute pHisoDerm ® (1 tablespoon to 10 tablespoons of water) or rubbing alcohol. Then snip off the dewclaws.

Bleeding: If there is bleeding, sprinkle a few grains of potassium permanganate (available from drugstores) over the area.

Removal of dewclaws in adult dogs: See a vet for surgery.

Note: Some show breeds require dewclaws. Owners of pedigreed dogs should consult breed standards.

Dislocations

Dislocations occur when a bone has become displaced (pulled away) from the joint. They should not be confused with a fracture, which is a broken bone; and unlike fractures, most dislocations should not be splinted.

Symptoms: While a fractured limb tends to swing freely, the dislocated limb is more rigid. There is usually pain and swelling around the dislocated joint and the leg may point in an odd direction, especially with dislocated elbows. The dog may attempt to walk on the dislocated leg, and the leg may support some of the weight before giving way.

Treatment: Do not bandage dislocated limbs; no support is necessary. Contact your vet as soon as possible.

Dislocated hip joint: If a dislocated hip cannot be corrected in four to six weeks, a false joint will develop and will work almost as well as the original. (A false joint is one created when the muscles around the hip become fibrous and thickened and able to support the joint.)

Feet

Dogs' feet are the equivalent of the soles of our shoes. But while leather soles wear out, dogs' feet do not. The pads are constantly growing and being resoled with dead, horny skin. Exceptions to this natural process occur after severe or prolonged exercise on very rough terrain, or after an injury in which the bottom of the pad has been sliced off.

If the bottom of the pad has been sliced off, allow it to heal naturally. Bathing will only soften the new skin that is forming and delay healing.

Foreign Bodies in the Foot: Punctures

Foreign bodies in the foot pads are usually pieces of glass that cut the pad and work their way into the paw, or pieces of grit that have found their way into existing breaks.

Symptoms: Acute lameness; hobbling; the dog may chew at its foot. In later stages, the affected foot will be hot and swollen and the skin of the pad will be shiny. There may be pus coming from the hole caused by the foreign object.

Treatment: You will need an assistant to hold the dog while you operate. (See Restraint and Handling.) Examine the dog's foot carefully under a bright light. Sterilize a needle by boiling it for twenty minutes, then carefully probe the hole until the foreign object is visible. With the aid of tweezers, remove it. Dress the wound. Use the same technique you would for removing a splinter from your own foot.

If probing with the needle does not remove the foreign body, prepare a kaolin poultice and apply it to the affected pad for two days. This should draw out the object, or at least make it easier for you to remove it with your needle and tweezers.

Heavy kaolin poultice: Heavy kaolin is a clay found in the hills of North Dakota, and sold in most drugstores.

Prepare the poultice by heating the kaolin clay and pouring it onto a wad of absorbent cotton. Do not apply it if it is too hot. Judge this by applying it to the back of your own hand. It should be very hot but not so hot that it burns you. Then bandage it around the foot for three or four hours, and repeat. (See Bandaging the Leg.) Use lots of adhesive when bandaging to prevent the dog from chewing it off. But if the animal still insists on chewing at it, use an Elizabethan collar. (See Elizabethan Collar.)

Interdigital Cyst

A distressing condition often seen in Alsatians, boxers, Labradors, and some terriers. Its cause is unknown.

Symptoms: A shiny, red swelling between the toes. This swelling is sore and painful and continues to swell until it bursts, liberating a clear, reddish fluid.

Treatment: Soften the affected part by bathing it four times a day in warm saline solution until the swelling bursts. (Saline solution is made by adding 1 teaspoon salt to 1 pint boiling water; allow the water to cool to body temperature before using). If the dog will not allow you to hold its foot in the solution, soak a clean cloth in it and bathe the foot. Paint the area with a solution of 2% carbolic acid (available at drugstores), using an eyedropper or paintbrush. Be careful not to use too much as it is caustic and painful.

In very serious cases, surgical treatment and a course of antibiotics may be necessary.

Lameness

In cases of severe lameness, the dog owner should not rely upon his own diagnosis if professional help is available. Improperly diagnosed fractures and dislocations can lead to severe complications. (See Fractures: General.)

Causes: As a general rule, in diagnosing causes of sudden lameness: (1) If the dog is severely lame and the limb is free-swinging, then the leg is probably fractured. (2) If there is displacement, that is, if the leg is not in its normal position, the leg may be dislocated. (3) If the affected limb is neither free-swinging nor displaced, a strain or sprain may be suspected. (4) A cut or foreign body (e.g., piece of glass, splinter) will also cause lameness.

More gradual and more permanent forms of lameness may be encountered in the elderly dog, caused by arthritis or neoplasms (cancerous growths). In such cases, simple analgesics may help.

Treatment: If the lameness persists for more than a few days, consult a veterinarian. It may be possible to cure the condition by surgical treatment, or, if the condition is inoperable, the vet may prescribe painkillers.

Limping

Causes: There are several possible causes for limping in dogs. If the cause is in the foot, the dog may lick the offending paw. Get the dog into a good light and carefully examine the paw for a thorn, tack, or small cut. You will find that it is easier to do this when the paw is wet; then the hair lies flat and the thorn or cut is more readily seen.

If it is not a thorn or a cut that is causing the limp, look for a cracked pad. You may not be able to see the cracks, so palpate the pad with your thumb. A cracked pad is very sensitive and pressure is painful, so be very gentle.

Next, check for a broken nail. If that is what is making the dog limp, a bit of adhesive tape around the broken nail will help until the nail grows back.

If none of these causes is evident, the limp may be the

result of a sprain. If it is a sprain, there will be swelling, pain, and local heat.

In an elderly dog, if there is no evidence of a sprain or injury to the paw, the limp may be caused by arthritis. To decide whether or not it is arthritis, observe the dog for a few days, and attempt to answer these questions: (1) Does the dog have difficulty in rising in the morning? Does it move more easily later in the day? (2) Does a change in the weather bring a variation in the lameness? (3) Is the dog unable to jump up, manage stairs? (4) Is it lame at a walk? At a gallop? (5) Is the lameness worse with exercise? (6) Is the lameness intermittent?

Treatment: If you cannot cure the lameness yourself, and you have to bring the dog to a vet, these are the questions he will ask you. Intelligent answers will greatly facilitate his treatment. (See Cuts; Wounds; Cracked Pads; Sprains and Strains; Fractures: General.)

Rickets

Symptoms: This disease affects young dogs from three weeks to six months of age. The first sign is usually a noticeable swelling of the wrist joint. Swellings will also be observed along the side of the chest. Severe cases will eventually develop bending of the long leg bones, causing bowleggedness.

Causes: Rickets is the result of calcium, phosphorus and vitamin D deficiencies.

Treatment: Administer bone flour (available from pet stores): 1 teaspoon per day for small dogs, up to 2 tablespoons per day for large dogs, for at least two months. Give vitamin A and vitamin D drops: 2 to 3 drops daily. Administration of cod-liver oil is not recommended for young dogs suffering from rickets, since it can alter the calcium to phosphorus ratio in the bones if given in excess of 2 drops daily.

Sprains and Strains

Sprains and strains are very similar in their effects and symptoms. A sprain involves the ligaments around a joint. A strain involves muscles. In both cases, the tissues are torn.

Causes: Sprains and strains are usually caused by violent exercise.

Symptoms: The diagnosis must often be made as the result of negative findings for fractures and dislocations. After these have been eliminated as the cause of the dog's lameness, look for a slight swelling around the joint or muscle.

Treatment: Alternate hot and cold compresses over the swelling until it goes down. If the animal is very uncomfortable, administer an analgesic.

Tar on the Feet

An occasional nuisance for owners of adventurous dogs.

Treatment: Stand the dog in a dishpan of warm saltwater with olive oil added. Whatever tar does not wash off during the foot bath should come off when you dry the dog's feet with a rag. If all the tar does not come off after the first washing and drying, repeat the process.

9

Problems of
the Back

Broken Back (Fractured Spine)

Fractures and dislocations of the spinal column are usually the result of some traumatic incident (e.g., an auto accident, a fall, or a blow with a stick across the back).

Symptoms: Generally, if the dog has been involved in an accident and cannot move both hind legs, and if there is no response when the toe is firmly pinched, it is logical to assume that the animal has a break or fracture of the spine. The dog usually lies with its front legs extended, and it is insensitive to pain below the affected portion of the spine. Urinary and fecal incontinence or retention are present.

These same symptoms could also indicate a slipped disk. But the slipped disk occurs spontaneously, not as the result of a traumatic incident.

Treatment: If the dog has been hit by a car, do not move it unless it is absolutely necessary. Telephone a vet, the police, or the A.S.P.C.A. If you are unable to do any of these things, use the backseat of a car as a stretcher, or get a board large enough to place the injured animal on, then slide the dog onto it very gently. Do not lift the dog. Tie the dog onto the board by wrapping a bandage around the dog and the board. Now lift the board and place it across the backseat of the car or on the floor if there is room, and drive to the nearest vet.

Prognosis: The outlook for dogs which suffer fractures and dislocations of the spine is not very hopeful. In the majority of cases, the dog will have to be put to sleep.

Broken Tail

Fractures of the tail occur after accidents, and in overenthusiastic dogs confined to small areas.

Fractures at root of tail: If the break occurs at the root of the tail, the full length of the tail will hang straight down. There will be pain and swelling at the fracture site.

Treatment: The dog owner should not attempt to treat root fractures. Professional assistance is necessary. If the animal is in pain, administer one to four 5-grain aspirin tablets, depending on the size of the dog. Then get the dog to a vet. (See How to Administer Tablets and Pills.)

Fractures along length of tail: Fractures of this type are easily identified: the dog can move its tail up to the fracture site, while the portion of the tail beyond the fracture hangs limp.

Treatment: If there is a delay of more than twenty-four hours before the dog can be seen by a vet, apply an adhesive tape dressing to support the length of the damaged tail.

Tape the break, tightly enough to provide support but not so tight that the circulation is cut off.

Fractures of tip of tail: Again, an adhesive tape dressing taped around the fracture; again, be careful not to tape it too tightly. Leave the dressing on until the fracture mends. It usually takes about three weeks for a tail fracture to heal.

Dogs with fractures, or suspected fractures, of the tail should be examined by a vet. Nerve damage often results, and that portion of the tail beyond the fracture may then have to be removed surgically.

Slipped Disk

This painful condition of the spine is fairly common in dogs with long bodies and short legs, such as dachshunds and corgis, but instances of it do occur in all breeds.

Causes: Breed failing, obesity. Also occurs in dogs which are violently overexercised.

Symptoms: Acute pain, especially when the dog attempts to walk. In severe cases, the dog cannot move its legs.

There may be rigidity or tenseness of the abdomen. Touch the dog's stomach lightly. The skin will be as tight as a drum. There may be retention of urine and feces, at first. Then, as the bladder and small intestine fill up the animal is unable to control itself and there is involuntary passage of the body wastes.

Treatment: The first thing to do is to ease the dog's pain. Administer one 5-grain aspirin tablet for small dogs, up to 25 grains for large dogs, once every twenty-four hours. (See How to Administer Tablets and Pills.)

The severity of the symptoms indicates the severity of the condition and while most mild instances of a slipped disk will right themselves, a vet should be consulted. If the condition persists or recurs frequently, surgery may be necessary.

10

Problems Affecting the Whole Body

Allergies: General (See Eczema)

An allergy is a reaction by the body to various substances to which it has become sensitized by previous exposure.

Causes: These substances include animal hair, plant pollen, certain drugs, certain foods, detergents and, often, the saliva of fleas.

Symptoms: Vomiting; diarrhea; dribbling; running eyes; red and itching skin; lumps on the skin; swelling of the face, lips, and eyelids.

Treatment: The best way of treating an allergy is, of course, to remove the cause. In situations where this is not possible, either because the allergic substance cannot be identified or because it is in the air (e.g., pollen), it will be necessary to treat the allergic dog with an appropriate drug. Most allergies respond well to antihistamines and corticosteroids. But the treatment must be given by a vet.

Anemia

A blood condition in which the oxygen-carrying capacity of the blood is reduced.

Causes: Loss of blood; red cell destruction (due to infection); poor blood formation (e.g., iron deficiency).

Symptoms: Lethargy; rapid pulse; unnatural paleness around the eyes, nose, and gums.

The symptoms and their degree vary with the situation. For example, a dog suffering from a debilitating disease will develop this unnatural pallor gradually, while a dog suffering from a hemorrhaging gastric ulcer will suddenly become very pale around the mucous membranes. (See Shock.)

Treatment: All anemic animals need professional treatment, since anemia is almost always symptomatic of other diseases or deficiencies (e.g., heartworm).

If chronic anemia is suspected and professional help is not available, administer ferrous sulfate tablets (obtainable at drugstores) until you can have your dog examined by a vet. Dosage: one 30 mg. tablet per day for small dogs, up to 90 mg. for large dogs. (See Body Weight; How to Administer Tablets and Pills.)

Breed Failings

A breed failing is an inherited physical defect and is due mainly to indiscriminate mating of a faulty stock.

To some extent, hereditary diseases and failings are found in all breeds, but some are seen more frequently in certain breeds.

Hip dysplasia: A hereditary condition of the hip joint

that causes lameness: Alsatians; Samoyeds; retrievers, Labrador and golden; or any large breed.

Patella luxation: Dislocation of the kneecap: cairns; Pekingese; poodles; Yorkshire terriers.

Entropion: Turned-in eyelids: spaniels; chow chows; retrievers; boxers; poodles.

Progressive retinal atrophy (PRA): A hereditary condition of the eyes leading to blindness: poodles; retrievers; spaniels.

Prolonged soft palate: Causes rattling in the throat: Bulldogs; pugs; Pekingese; boxers.

Labial eczema: Eczema of the lips: King Charles spaniels; Irish setters.

Luxation of the eye lens: Lens slipping out of place: wire-haired fox terriers; Staffordshire bull terriers.

Calcium Deficiency

The main function of calcium in the diet is to aid the growth and formation of teeth and bones. Proper amounts of calcium in the diet of puppies are essential. A lack of calcium in the diet will cause ricketlike changes: swollen, tender joints, arched back, and stiff legs. Acute calcium deficiency in the lactating dog will produce a condition called milk fever. (See Milk Fever.)

Although milk is a natural source of calcium, a dog suffering from a calcium deficiency needs a concentrated dose and should drink a solution made with calcium gluconate powder (available from drugstores). Add 4 tablespoons of the powder to ½ pint of water. Since the dog will probably refuse to drink this voluntarily, the owner should be prepared to force-feed. (See Nutrition; Force Feeding.)

Canine Infectious Hepatitis

A highly contagious viral infection transmittable only to other dogs. Unlike distemper, this form of virus has a low mortality rate. The disease exists in four well-defined forms (worst first):

Fatal fulminating form: This form causes sudden death, after a rapid collapse which may be preceded by blood-stained diarrhea.

Acute form: The dog looks "poorly" for four to six hours; animal is depressed; may have high temperature; may vomit blood; has bloodstained diarrhea. After about six hours, if not professionally treated, the dog may fall into a coma and die.

Treatment: Get the dog to the vet before the coma stage, and there is a chance that its life may be saved.

Subacute nonfatal form: The dog's temperature is around 105° F.; rapid heartbeat; swollen, inflamed tonsils; bloodstained diarrhea; yellowing of eyes and gums (jaundice).

Prognosis: Occasionally death does occur, but if the animal survives the first forty-eight hours, it will not die.

Subclinical form: In this form, there are no definite symptoms. The dog is simply out of condition: lethargic with little appetite. A blood test is the only way of making a definite diagnosis.

Treatment: Professional help must be sought. The dog owner can only treat the symptoms as they arise, and often they pass unnoticed.

Administer vitamin B complex tablets: 2 tablets once a day for small dogs, up to 5 tablets twice a day for large dogs, for two weeks. Also give vitamin B_{12} tablets: 2 tablets twice a day for small dogs, up to 10 tablets twice a day for large dogs, for two weeks. These vitamins are helpful as a supplement to professional medical treatment. (See Technique for Administering Tablets and Pills.)

Chorea (St. Vitus' Dance)

Symptoms: Pronounced and frequent twitching of a muscle or muscles, especially of the face and legs. Also, a clicking of the jaw. Often seen as the sequel to distemper.

Treatment: There is no known remedy for this condition. Fortunately, in mild cases, it does not trouble the dog and is not transmitted through breeding.

Diabetes Insipidus (Drinking Diabetes)

A disease of the pituitary gland.

Symptoms: Increased thirst (be sure to keep the dog's water bowl full); frequent, pale-colored urination. There is no smell of acetone on the breath. Laboratory tests will show no sugar in the urine. (See also Chronic Interstitial Nephritis.)

Treatment: The vet may put the dog on a course of hormone treatment.

Diabetes Mellitus (Sugar Diabetes)

Cause: Diabetes is a chronic disorder in which there is an abnormal amount of sugar in the blood and urine caused by a malfunctioning pancreas.

Symptoms: Increased appetite; increased thirst, frequent urination; traces of sugar in the urine; a sweetish odor of acetone (like nail polish remover) on the dog's breath. There may be loss of weight. Secondary symptoms of cataracts may appear in the eyes. If untreated, the animal may fall into a diabetic coma. (See Unconsciousness.) A definite diagnosis must be made by a vet, after analysis of a urine sample. (See Taking Samples of Feces and Urine.)

Treatment: Home treatment, after professional consultation, usually consists of daily injections of insulin. (See How to Give an Injection.) The drug should always be given before feeding.

Overdose: If an accidental overdose of insulin is administered, insulin coma will follow. This condition can be reversed by giving glucose or sugar by mouth.

Distemper Complex (Distemper and Hard Pad)

Distemper is caused by a virus. It is highly contagious and infectious, and any dog suspected of having distemper should be kept away from other animals. Dogs of all ages are susceptible. The incubation period is three to fifteen days.

Vaccination: Dogs should be first vaccinated at the age of ten weeks. Since the immunity produced by distemper vaccination lasts for about a year, an annual booster shot is recommended.

Symptoms: Depression and lethargy; loss of appetite; very high temperature (105° F.). There is a watery discharge from the eyes and nose. Later it becomes yellow and sticky. The dog develops a dry cough. At this stage the dog's temperature begins to fluctuate from 104° F. to normal (around 101°).

Conjunctivitis develops. (Conjunctivitis is an inflammation of the membranes around the eye.)

The nasal discharge dries into a hard greenish-yellow scab, and there is evidence of tonsillitis, possibly vomiting, definitely diarrhea.

Second stage: Two or three weeks after the onset of the disease, the nervous symptoms appear. These may take the form of convulsions, or of twitching of muscles on the dog's face and on the forelegs. Circling may occur. The dog runs around and around. This stage may be associated with blindness and aimless wandering.

Treatment: Professional help must be obtained. The treatment will depend entirely on the stage of the disease. The only treatment the owner can give is empirical, that is, to treat any symptoms as they arise.

Since distemper is a viral infection, antibiotics cannot help to cure it. They can only prevent secondary bacterial infections. The vet will treat the disease with other more specific and sophisticated drugs, but an early diagnosis must be made.

The success of any treatment for distemper depends largely upon the early identification of the disease. The later it is recognized, the less optimistic the prognosis.

Hard Pad: Hard pad is not really a separate entity. It is another example of how complex a viral infection can be.

Symptoms: Hard pad has the same symptoms as distemper, with the addition of: severe diarrhea; hardening of the foot pads and the nose, occurring about fifteen days after onset of the infection.

Treatment: Again, the success of the vet's treatment

depends mainly on how quickly the dog owner realizes that his pet is ill.

Drowning

Treatment: Get the dog out of the water. If the animal is unconscious, lay it on its side and open its mouth; make sure that its tongue is out and that there is nothing obstructing the windpipe. Use your finger to check for grass, sand, mud, etc., in the dog's mouth.

If the dog is still unconscious, lift it by its hind legs and allow the water to drain out of its mouth. Administer artificial respiration or mouth-to-mouth resuscitation, which is slightly more effective. (See Artificial Respiration.)

Electric Shock

Usually caused by the dog's chewing on an electric cord. So, if you find your dog lying unconscious next to a badly frayed electric cord, you will know to treat it for electric shock.

Warning: Be careful! Often a shocked dog urinates, and the pool of urine makes an excellent conductor. Do not step into it, and do not touch the dog until you have turned off the current, or you will need someone to give *you* first aid.

If you are unable to turn off the electricity, put on a rubber glove or grab a thick, dry towel and pull the electric plug out of the outlet. Or, get a wooden stick such as a broom handle and push the animal out of the urine and away from the electric cord.

Treatment: If the dog has not regained consciousness by

this time, administer artificial respiration. If the dog is small enough, try swinging first. (See Artificial Respiration.)

Excessive Thirst (Drink-Vomit Cycle)

Symptoms: Increased thirst is a symptom of several conditions, all of them serious (see *Note* below). Since the average dog owner is not competent to make a diagnosis, follow these general rules until a vet can examine the animal.

Treatment: Never withhold water from a dog with excessive thirst, unless the dog is vomiting. When a dog starts on the drink-vomit cycle, it will continue drinking and then vomiting until dehydration and death occur.

To break the cycle, withhold all water for twelve hours. Then give the dog 1 or 2 tablespoons (depending upon size) of a water and glucose mixture, every two hours for the next twelve hours. The mixture should consist of 3–4 tablespoons glucose dissolved in 1 pint water. (If glucose is not readily available, an ice cube may be given every hour.)

If the dog is still vomiting after twelve hours, seek professional help.

Note: Possible causes of greatly increased thirst are: diabetes; chronic interstitial nephritis; pyometra; increased body temperature; poisoning; enteritis; gastritis; other infections.

Fits (Convulsions)

Causes: The cause of a fit cannot be diagnosed from the type of fit or its severity.

A fit can be the result of a variety of causes, such as epilepsy, a virus, worms, teething, or the sequel to a very high fever. In very young puppies, it could have been caused by something as simple as overexcitement.

Symptoms: Fits take several forms, all of them violent and frightening. The fit usually begins with the dog shaking its head. This is followed by champing of the jaws, salivation, incoordination, screaming, and the involuntary passage of urine and feces. Then, the dog may fall on its side and make running movements. The action of the jaws converts the saliva into a viscid froth, causing the dog to foam at the mouth and often terrifying those who should be helping the animal.

Treatment: The only thing you can do for a dog which is having a fit is prevent it from hurting itself. First, make sure that it does not hurt you. Remember, the most affectionate pet becomes a dangerous animal during a fit. Do not try to calm it by petting or stroking. It will not do your dog any good. You will just be bitten. Do not waste time talking to the dog; it cannot hear you.

Get some blankets or pillows and throw them into a closet or small room without furniture or sharp corners. If possible, darken the room. Then, move the dog into the padded area.

Technique for moving large dogs: Get behind the dog. Grab it firmly by the skin of the neck, just behind the head, with one hand on either side. Drag the dog to the padded room or closet, put it inside and close the door. Check in ten minutes to see if the fit has passed and if you can safely get the animal to the vet.

Technique for moving smaller, more agile dogs: Get behind the dog. Grab the scruff of the neck with one hand.

With your other hand, grab both of the dog's back legs and stretch them.

Once the animal is in a safe room, leave it alone. The fit will pass. It may take five minutes, it could take thirty, but eventually the fit will pass. When it does, allow the dog to rest quietly.

Further treatment will depend upon the cause of the fit. Without medical training one can only make a guess, not a diagnosis. Seek professional help if possible.

FRACTURES

A fracture is the term used to describe a broken bone.

Simple fracture: If only the bone is broken and there is no communicating wound between the fracture and the skin, it is called a simple fracture.

Compound fracture: If the skin over the fracture site is broken and bone protrudes, making it possible for germs to enter from the external wound, it is called a compound fracture.

Complicated fracture: This type of fracture may be either simple or compound, but there is also injury to some internal organ, blood vessel, nerve, or joint.

An originally simple fracture can be turned into a compound or complicated fracture by allowing the injured animal complete freedom of movement, or by carelessness or ignorance on the part of the owner.

When rendering first aid for fractures, there are two main objectives: to guard against further injury, and to reduce the dog's pain.

Causes: Most fractures are caused by accidents, but

occasionally they occur spontaneously when a bone is undergoing pathological change (e.g., in calcium deficiency or in bone cancer).

Symptoms: The fractures most commonly seen in dogs are fractures involving the legs. There is acute and profound lameness of the affected leg; considerable pain; possible swelling at the fracture site; possible shortening of the fractured limb. When the dog is lifted off the ground, the affected limb will swing freely but abnormally. Generally some or all of these symptoms can be seen in a dog with a leg fracture.

General treatment: Injured dogs must be approached and handled with great caution. An animal in pain is dangerous to you and to itself. (See Restraint and Handling). If a fracture is suspected, handle the limb or broken bone as little as possible. Make the dog as comfortable and as warm as possible. Administer aspirin to control the pain: 5 grains for a small dog, up to 25 grains for a large dog. Administer once only. (See How to Administer Tablets and Pills.)

Basic first aid is aimed at providing a support for the fractured bone. To accomplish this a splint is applied to the fractured bone at the point of the fracture. The splint serves as a vice between which the broken bones are held in place until professional help can be obtained.

Do not attempt to straighten or reset broken bones in the correct position. This will cause extreme pain and should be done only under anesthetic. Seek professional assistance as soon as possible. Splints applied by dog owners must be considered as temporary measures and should be attempted only when a vet is not available. (See instructions for making a splint under Fractures of the Limbs.)

Fractures of the Upper Parts of the Limbs

These are extremely difficult to splint and should be left alone until professional help is available.

Treatment: Large dogs with fractured limbs will be able to hobble into a car for transportation to the vet. Small dogs should be carried with fractured limb outermost. For example, if the left leg is fractured, carry the dog on its right side.

Fractures of the Lower Parts of the Limbs

These are among the most common fractures seen. The dog will be unable to put the injured foot on the ground and, as it hobbles along, the leg will swing freely.

Treatment: If professional help is not available within twenty-four hours, fractures of the lower leg should be supported by a simple splint.

To make a splint: First tie a tape muzzle around the dog's mouth. (See Restraint and Handling.) Lay the dog on its side, injured leg uppermost. Then place the injured leg on a thin piece of wood, or corrugated cardboard, and tape the leg to the wood with strips of adhesive tape.

This splint is intended simply to prevent excessive movement and not as a permanent repair, or as a substitute for a vet's services.

Fractures of the Bones of the Foot

A fractured foot will be very swollen, very sore, and

may have a number of cuts on it. The dog must be seen by a vet. If one is not immediately available, apply a bandage as already described. (See Bandaging the Leg.) Get professional help at the first opportunity.

Fractures of the Jaws

Causes: Fractures of the jaws are frequently seen in dogs hit by cars or dogs which have fallen from a considerable height. When a dog falls from a height, the front legs give way and the chin hits the ground, causing a fracture of the lower jaw.

If the dog falls from an even greater height, there may be a fracture of the upper jaw, which appears as a split in the roof of the mouth.

Symptoms: If the lower jaw has been fractured, it usually hangs slightly open. This is accompanied by profuse salivation, dribbling, and drooling. Closer examination will reveal a pronounced split in the middle of the front teeth, or a split in the middle of the mouth if the upper jaw is fractured.

Treatment: If the jaw is hanging open, tie a light dressing under the chin and around the back of the head (tie the dressing off behind the ears) to give support to the jaw. Then, get the injured dog to a vet.

Fractures of the Pelvis

Symptoms: A dog with a fractured pelvis will be unable to support any weight on either of its hind legs. However, since a dog with both hind legs fractured or with a spinal fracture will also be unable to stand, a definite diagnosis of a fractured pelvis can only be made by means of an X ray.

Treatment: A fracture of the pelvis does not require splinting. Keep the dog in a confined space until a vet has been consulted.

Fractures of the Skull

Causes: Seen after road accidents, falls, blows. They may cause incoordination, unconsciousness, or nosebleeds. Fractures of the skull can only be definitely diagnosed by X ray. If a skull fracture is suspected, do not bandage the skull; it may be a depressed fracture and bandaging will only make it worse.

Treatment: Use simple first aid to stop any bleeding. Be very gentle, especially in the area of the skull. Give no drugs or fluids until a vet is seen.

Gangrene

The term applies to either a specific localized condition, such as an infection, or a portion of the body in which the tissues are dead because the blood supply to that portion of the body has been restricted.

Infection: When gangrene is due to an infection, it usually follows bite wounds, especially on the feet. If the infection is left untreated, it may become gangrenous. A bite around the wrist area can become infected, and the blockage of the blood vessels causes gangrene of the toes.

The infection develops fairly rapidly and the infected area becomes swollen, foul-smelling, and gives off a bubbly discharge.

Treatment: None that the nonprofessional can administer. Get the dog to a vet.

Blood restriction: Gangrene caused by restriction of the blood supply to a part of the body is seen when bandages are applied too tightly or when a tourniquet is left on too long.

It also occurs (far too frequently) when children put rubber bands around the dog's neck, paws, or scrotum. When the restricting band is on the neck, the gangrene occurs under the band; on the paws and scrotum, the gangrene appears on the parts themselves.

Treatment: Remove the source of constriction. Clean the area with hydrogen peroxide, or soap and water, and apply warm compresses to encourage the blood to circulate again. Get professional help.

Grass Seeds

In the summer and early autumn, the drying seeds of barley grasses can cause a good deal of pain by penetrating between the dog's toes, down its ears, into its eyes, or up its nose. If left untreated the seeds, which are barbed like fishhooks, will migrate inward, eventually producing discharging wounds.

Symptoms:

Ears: A grass seed down the ear causes very painful symptoms. The dog rubs its face on the ground, paws at its ears, and walks with its head on one side as though attempting to dislodge something.

Nose: A grass seed up the nose will cause severe sneezing bouts.

Eyes: Profuse crying from one eye only. Extreme irritation of the eye. It will become very red and obviously painful.

Between the toes: A grass seed lodged between the toes produces pustules which may cause the dog to limp. If left untreated, the seed will work its way into the foot and produce breaks in the skin that may be confused with those of interdigital cysts.

Treatment:

Ears: Pour warm olive oil or cooking oil into the ear, and massage the ear gently to float the seeds out.

Nose: Get a good light and shine it up the dog's nose. If the seed is visible, it may be removed with tweezers. If you do use tweezers, be very careful not to injure the delicate nasal lining.

If your dog is difficult to control, you will need an assistant to hold the animal. (See Restraint and Handling.) And if the dog is very difficult, don't attempt to put anything up its nose. Leave treatment to the vet.

Eyes: If the seed has not penetrated the eyeball, wash it out of the eye with a saline solution. (Add 1 teaspoon salt to 1 pint boiling water, and allow the solution to cool.) If the seed has penetrated the eyeball, do not attempt to remove it; get the dog to a vet.

Between the toes: If you can see the seed, use a pair of tweezers to pull it out.

Growths, Tumors, Cancers

Tumors or cancers can affect any organ, system, or part

of the body at any age. They are divided into two groups: benign and malignant.

Benign tumors: Grow slowly; clearly defined, round lumps; cool to the touch; do not spread to other parts of the body.

Malignant tumors: Grow rapidly; not clearly defined, and it is sometimes difficult to tell where the tumor ends and the healthy part of the body begins. They are warm to the touch; spread to other parts of the body; tend to ulcerate; and if left untreated, will eventually kill.

Any swelling could be a tumor and should be examined by a vet immediately. Some malignant tumors can be stopped if they are caught early.

Heat Stroke

Cause: Prolonged exposure to a source of heat, or over-crowding. Classic cases of heat stroke occur when dogs are left in cars on hot days or packed into traveling cages that are too small for them.

Breeds with heavy coats are particularly susceptible to heat stroke, and the condition is aggravated by lack of water.

Symptoms: Panting; dullness; stumbling; sweating through the foot pads.

In the later stages the dog runs a very high temperature, up to 110° F., falls into a coma and finally dies.

Treatment: Give the dog water immediately. Cool the animal by hosing and sponging with cold water and by applying ice packs all over its body, with special attention to the head and chest. Administer a glucose and water solution: 4 tablespoons glucose to 1 pint water; ¼ pint for small dogs, up to 1 pint for large dogs.

Hysteria

Certain individual dogs and certain breeds seem to be hysteria-prone.

Hysteria usually begins with a long bout of barking. The dog acts terrified, and runs about yelping wildly and bouncing off walls and furniture. As with fits, there may be involuntary passage of urine and feces. The hysterical dog will not respond to commands. It will try to evade capture and will bite if it can. Handle it carefully. (See Restraint and Handling.)

Treatment: Treat a hysterical dog as you would treat a dog having a fit (See Fits.) or convulsions. Get it into a quiet, darkened, empty room or closet where it cannot hurt itself.

The line between hysteria and a fit is very thin, and if not promptly attended to, a hysterical dog may drift over that line and into a full-fledged fit.

Leptospirosis

This is a bacterial disease and not due to a virus. It may respond to specific antibiotic therapy once the disease has been identified. The incubation period is five to fifteen days.

Cause: Mainly, the infection comes from contact with infected urine, which is why puppies of both sexes and male dogs catch leptospirosis far more often than bitches, which tend to be more discreet in their urinating habits.

Symptoms: Loss of appetite; excessive thirst; lethargy; fever as high as 106°F.; sore abdomen; severe diarrhea; vomiting; sore, red eyes. The dog moves slowly with evident pain and may show signs of jaundice—its eyes, gums, and tongue may have a yellowish cast.

Treatment: Get professional treatment, if at all possible. The specific drug for this condition is streptomycin, which must be given by a vet.

The only home treatment is to deal with the symptoms as they arise. These symptoms include thirst, diarrhea, and vomiting. (See Excessive Thirst.)

Good hygiene is essential. Wash your hands after touching the dog. Keep the dog out of the room in which you eat. Sprinkle disinfectant in or around your home wherever the dog urinates. Owners must not forget that they and their family can catch this disease from the dog and must act accordingly.

Prognosis: If the disease is recognized and treatment begun early, there is an excellent chance of recovery. Once jaundice has set in, however, the outlook is less optimistic.

Warning: This disease is highly contagious and can be transmitted from dogs to people.

Lightning

Dogs taking shelter under trees or in close contact with metallic objects are occasionally struck by lightning.

Symptoms: The dog may be burned and may also show signs of shock, such as incoordination or even paralysis.

Treatment: Treat for shock by keeping the dog warm and quiet, then treat the burns. (See Burns and Scalds; Shock.) Administer a simple stimulant, such as strong, cooled black coffee or tea. Also give a mixture of 4 tablespoons glucose to 1 pint water. (See Force-Feeding.) Seek professional help.

Motion Sickness (Airsickness, Car Sickness, Seasickness)

This condition is common in dogs, especially those unaccustomed to traveling.

Symptoms: Restlessness; excessive salivation; persistent vomiting.

Treatment: Before the trip, visit the vet, who will administer an animal tranquilizer. If animal tranquilizers are not available, preparations for human travel sickness, available at the drugstore without prescription, may be administered instead. The dosage will vary with the size of the dog, but a fair estimate is one-quarter of the adult human dosage per 20 pounds animal body weight.

Prevention: Before long journeys, withhold all food for twenty-four hours, but give the dog plenty of water.

Get the dog accustomed to car travel by taking it on short trips when possible. Also, allow the dog to spend time in the car when it is not in use.

Neuralgia (Nerve Pain)

Symptoms: Sudden and obvious pain; tense muscles in the dog's neck, back, or legs. These attacks of neuralgia are intermittent and may last for several hours.

Treatment: Keep the dog warm and allow it to rest. An infrared ray lamp is a great comfort to a dog suffering from neuralgia. Mount the lamp about three feet over the dog's bed and leave it on all night. An electric blanket or hot water bottle may be substituted for the lamp. Administer up to two 5-grain aspirin tablets, depending upon body weight, to ease the pain.

Pain

Symptoms: Dogs show pain by abnormal behavior or by assuming abnormal positions. There is no register for pain. The owner must observe his dog's reactions as a guide to the location and severity of the pain.

Pain in different parts of the body produces different reactions. For example: pain in the legs causes lameness; pain in the abdomen causes restlessness, sitting or lying in abnormal positions, and whining. There is also a tendency to seek out cold places, such as cement floors, to lie on. Pain in the head causes languor or restlessness, or both, alternately. The dog paws its head and presses its head against the wall. Acute pain causes the dog to cry, whine, whimper, and act frightened. The dog will look at or lick the affected area.

Treatment: A dog manifesting symptoms of pain should be carefully observed for a moment. Its behavior may give you a clue to the problem. For example, a dog with a foreign body in its paw will chew at its foot, while a dog with a foreign body in its mouth will paw at its mouth.

After locating the site of the pain, examine it carefully with the aid of a good light. Don't let your dog's pain panic you. If you can observe and trace its cause, you may be able to alleviate it.

Rabies

Although rabies usually occurs in bats, dogs, foxes, and skunks, all warm-blooded animals—including man—are susceptible.

Cause: A virus infection which is transmitted by an

infected animal biting another animal. The incubation period varies from fifteen days to several months.

Symptoms: The symptoms of rabies are easily confused with those of many other diseases. They include: a marked change in behavior (e.g., docile dogs become aggressive, aggressive dogs docile); vomiting and diarrhea. The dog often behaves as if it has a foreign body in its mouth, coughing, drooling, and pawing at its mouth. From one to three days after the onset of these symptoms, the affected dog will become vicious, biting and scratching at the slightest provocation. In the final stages, many dogs that are normally quite sociable will seek solitude.

Treatment: Treatment is given to any human being who may have been bitten. If one has been exposed to a dog who is suspected of being rabid, the animal should be confined but not killed, in order for a correct diagnosis to be made. If you are bitten by any stray animal, or if rabies is suspected, call a doctor at once.

Prevention: Beware of all strays. Have your dog vaccinated against rabies. If you have the slightest suspicion that your dog may be rabid, confine it, and notify a vet immediately.

Shock

Shock is the term used to describe a state of collapse characterized by an acute and progressive failure of the circulatory system.

Causes: While the exact causes of shock are unknown, the condition follows most forms of severe trauma caused by serious injuries, massive hemorrhages, heart failure, serious burns, and dehydration.

Symptoms: Apathy; low body temperature; pale skin,

gums, and tongue; rapid thready pulse; rapid shallow breathing; thirst; and, finally, complete collapse.

Treatment: Keep the dog warm by wrapping it in a blanket. Keep the dog quiet and get it to a vet. The prime form of treatment is to restore the amount of circulating fluid in the blood vessels through a transfusion, which can only be administered by a vet.

Trembling or Shivering

Causes: Dogs shiver when they are: frightened; cold; running a high fever; excited.

Treatment: Shivering or trembling that goes on for longer than half an hour is a sign that something is seriously amiss. Examine the dog for fever. (See Taking Temperature.)

Unconsciousness

When you find a dog unconscious, unless the cause is immediately apparent (e.g., a large, gaping chest wound), do not waste time searching for the cause. The only exception to this is when the animal has been in contact with an electric wire. (See Electric Shock.) The reasons why animals lose consciousness may be divided into two very general categories.

Primary causes: The dog loses consciousness as the result of a lesion affecting the nervous system and the brain. This occurs after car accidents or similar injuries, fits, strokes, and narcosis produced by poisoning.

Secondary causes: The dog loses consciousness as the

result of ailments affecting other areas of the body. These include diabetic coma, uremic coma (poison from the kidneys), calcium deficiency, shock, electric shock, drowning, and heart attack.

Treatment: If the dog does not appear to be breathing, do not assume that it is dead, unless certain other factors are valid. Even if you think the dog is dead, and you cannot detect breathing, give artificial respiration for at least thirty minutes unless rigor mortis is evident. (See Artificial Respiration.)

Fainting: Dogs faint if the blood supply to the brain is reduced or is deficient in oxygen. This occurs in dogs which are in a state of shock, or whose hearts are not functioning properly.

Treatment: Dogs that have fainted will recover spontaneously. Make sure the animal's tongue is out and that nothing is blocking the windpipe. Most dogs recover from faints in three or four minutes.

Vomiting

Causes: Infectious disease (e.g., distemper); acute abdomen (e.g., peritonitis, intestinal obstruction); indigestion (overeating); metabolic disorders (e.g., hepatitis or nephritis); administration of certain drugs (e.g., digitalis); nervous disorders (motion sickness, fear); pharyngeal irritation (e.g., tonsillitis); poisoning; parasites; hernias; tumors; inflammation of the gullet; toxemia.

Blood in Vomit

Causes: Fresh blood in your dog's vomit may be caused by accidents, tumors, or foreign bodies which have cut the mouth, throat, or gullet. If the blood found in the vomit is black, it comes from the stomach or from the small intestine, and may be caused by a stomach ulcer or by tumors.

Treatment: There is no home treatment for this condition, since it is not possible for the dog owner to diagnose the cause accurately.

As a temporary measure, the dog should not be fed until a vet has examined it. If the vet cannot be seen within twenty-four hours, give the dog a glucose and water solution: 4 ounces of glucose to 1 pint of water. Small dogs should be given ¼ pint, large dogs, 1 pint. Give once only in a twenty-four-hour period.

Drink-Vomit Cycle (See Excessive Thirst)

Vomiting Induced by Poisons

The group of poisons that cuase vomiting includes most of the common poisons such as arsenic, phosphorus, and decayed food.

Symptoms: Look for burns in the dog's mouth or on its tongue. The vomit will give off a pronounced acid smell.

Treatment: Administer corn oil to soothe the stomach lining: 4 ounces to 1 pint, depending upon size of dog. (See Force Feeding.)

Warning: Do not administer emetics to a dog that is already vomiting or is unconscious.

WEIGHT PROBLEMS

Excessive Appetite

Causes: A dramatic increase in appetite suggests: abdominal tumors; diseases that interfere with food absorption; fat deposits common in spayed and neutered animals; simple greed (may be the result of a neurotic condition or of brain damage); pregnancy.

Treatment: Depends on the cause. Abdominal tumors and food absorption diseases require professional treatment. In the case of desexed dogs, feed them less than they want. Simple greed is beyond the scope of treatment and the last cause treats itself.

Loss of Appetite (Anorexia)

It is not unusual for a dog to lose its appetite for twenty-four hours. But if the dog refuses food after twenty-four hours, consider this loss of appetite as a symptom of something else. Check for: generalized disease; tartar on the teeth; foreign body in the mouth or throat; sore mouth or sore throat. Look for sores in the mouth and red gums. Feel the animal's larynx. If it is sore, the dog will cough.

Treatment: Examine the dog's mouth and throat for obstructions. If there are none, take the dog's temperature. If the temperature is above normal, a vet should be consulted. If a vet is not available, try to tempt the dog's appetite with succulent taste treats such as boiled, deboned chicken, strong cheeses, or smoked salmon.

If the dog has still not eaten after forty-eight hours, consult a vet.

Weight Gain

Causes: A great increase in weight over a three to four week period is abnormal and suggests one of the following possibilities: abdominal tumor (see Index); fluid in the abdomen (some serious diseases produce large amounts of fluid in the abdomen); compulsive eating (may be the result of simple greed or brain damage); pregnancy; tendency of desexed dogs to put on weight; thyroid deficiency.

Treatment: This list is a general guide to the possible causes of a sudden weight increase in your dog. Proper diagnosis and treatment must be left to a vet.

Weight Loss

Causes: Sudden loss of weight may be caused by: reduced intake of food; persistent vomiting; reduced absorption of food; diseases such as chronic nephritis or hepatitis; diabetes mellitus; tumors; internal parasites.

Treatment: Try to identify the cause and remedy it. In the event of continuing weight loss, get professional assistance.

11

Problems of
Female Dogs Only

Abortion or Miscarriage

See Miscarriage or Abortion; Mating; Mismating.

Agalactia

Agalactia is the inability of an animal to give milk.

Causes: The cause can be hereditary; it can be the result of a hormonal imbalance or the sequel to an infection or breast cancer. Agalactia often occurs in bitches giving birth to their first litters.

Symptoms: The behavior of the puppies is your best indication of agalactia. If they are not getting their milk, they will scream and whine with hunger and will be restless and fretful, just as a human baby would be. The mother, however, will appear quite normal.

Treatment: Apply warm compresses to the mother's

mammary glands for ten minutes at a time, four to five times a day. Gently massage the mammary glands with olive oil to stimulate and restore their function. Hormone therapy with pituitary hormones, which requires the services of a vet, may induce milk production within twenty-four hours.

These treatments, of course, apply only to the mother. Meanwhile, while waiting for the production of milk, the newborn puppies must be fed every two hours. (See Orphan Puppies.)

Diet for Brood Bitch

A brood bitch is a bitch used for breeding.

Brood bitches may be fed their usual diet with extra milk and fat added. An extra pint of milk a day plus two egg yolks should be adequate. Also add one-half to two tablespoons of sterilized bone flour per day per 10 pounds body weight.

Do not feed the bitch biscuits from the day of mating until birth occurs. Dog biscuits, which contain carbohydrates, tend to make dogs fatter and a pregnant bitch should not be overweight.

False Pregnancy

This condition, to varying degrees, occurs in most bitches about nine weeks after the end of every heat period. It occurs because the ovaries of the female undergo the same changes as when mating and conception have taken place.

Symptoms: The symptoms of false pregnancy are exactly the same as those which occur during the final stages of a real pregnancy, with the exception of the abdominal enlargement (though this does occasionally occur). The mammary glands fill with milk. The bitch may try to make a bed or nest for herself. She may also start nursing woolly toys.

Treatment: Reassure and quiet her. Psychologically as well as physically, she is going through a difficult time. Milk sedation, or analgesics such as Lobak or Panadol, a 250 mg. tablet twice a day for small dogs, up to a 500 mg. tablet twice a day for large dogs, will ease the bitch's discomfort. (See How to Administer Tablets and Pills.)

Add a pinch of Epsom salts to her food during this period. This will help her get rid of the milk produced by the false pregnancy. (It may also cause a mild case of diarrhea for a day or so.)

Severe cases: Severe or persistent cases will require hormone treatment by a vet. If the case is very severe or recurs persistently, the owner should give the bitch canine contraceptive pills to suppress the heat or have her spayed. These pills may be obtained from a veterinarian.

Hemorrhage from the Vagina

While some slight bleeding from the vagina is normal during heat periods, heavy bleeding requires immediate professional assistance.

Treatment: Keep the bitch warm and quiet until professional help is available. (See Shock; Miscarriage or Abortion.)

Mating: Heat (Bitches)

"Heat" or "season" is the term used to describe the time when the female dog will mate. It is during this period that pregnancy may occur.

A bitch's first season usually occurs when she is between six and nine months old. Bitches are capable of conceiving throughout their lives. They are never too old to have a litter.

Bitches come into heat twice a year. This regular cyclic progression is interrupted only by pregnancy. Each heat lasts approximately eighteen days and may be divided into two stages.

First Stage: During the first stage the bitch's vulva swells noticeably and the owner will observe a blood-tinged discharge. The bitch becomes attractive to and attracts the attention of male dogs, but during this first stage she will not be interested in mating. Her appetite and drinking habits may become capricious. This stage lasts about nine days after the signs of heat first appear. Then the second stage begins.

Second stage: During this stage the bitch is capable of conceiving. The discharge from the vulva is straw-colored and free from blood. She will readily accept any male dog. She develops wanderlust and, if allowed, will stray from home in the company of male followers.

Successful breeding: An owner who wishes to breed his bitch should attempt to ensure that mating occurs as soon as possible after the bleeding stops. Successful breeding is most likely to occur ten to twelve days after the beginning of heat.

Control of heat: Very few owners want their bitches to

become pregnant with every heat. Fortunately, there are several methods available for preventing unwanted pregnancies.

Abortion (mismating): Accidental mating can be aborted within thirty-six hours, with an injection of stilbestrol given by a vet. This injection may bring the animal into heat for an additional twenty-one days.

Spaying (ovariohysterectomy): Removal of the uterus and ovaries to prevent heat. Its only drawback is that it is irreversible. However, it is preferable to an unwanted litter.

It is commonly and erroneously believed that a bitch will be healthier and happier if she has at least one litter before being spayed, or that it is cruel and unnatural to interfere with an animal's sex life. We suggest that owners who subscribe to these folk prejudices examine their attitudes to be sure that they are not confusing their own sexuality with that of their pets.

Contraceptive tablets: For the owner who does not wish to take the irreversible step of hysterectomy, but does not want litter after litter of puppies, there are contraceptive tablets available from vets that suppress or postpone heat. However, these contraceptive tablets are not suitable for every bitch. Consult a vet for further information regarding brand names and dosages.

Postcoital problems: After mating, the dog and the bitch may remain "tied" together for about twenty minutes. Well-meaning but uninformed owners may attempt to separate them by throwing a pail of cold water over them, or by pulling them apart. This can cause an uncontrollable hemorrhage of the dog's penis, as well as inflicting appreciable damage to the vagina. When a pair of dogs are tied together after mating, leave them alone until they separate.

Milk Fever (Eclampsia)

This condition is seen in all breeds of dogs but it occurs more frequently in the smaller breeds, especially those which have just had large litters.

Cause: Calcium deficiency.

Symptoms: Milk fever usually can be seen just before the puppies are weaned, about five to six weeks after birth. The bitch becomes very restless, whimpers a great deal and lies with her legs extended, breathing rapidly. She may lose her sense of coordination and fall over when she tries to stand. This stage is associated with a rise in body temperature, up to 107° F. There is dribbling, rigidity, and convulsions.

Warning: If the bitch in this state is left untreated she will die.

Treatment: Treatment is simple, but it must be administered by a vet. It consists of intravenous administration of calcium borogluconate. As interim treatment: if convulsions have not started, owners can mix 4 ounces calcium borogluconate (available at drugstores) with 1 pint water, and give this solution by mouth until the symptoms stop or the vet arrives. Give one 5-grain aspirin tablet per 20 pounds, up to 25 grains for large dogs. This may help to control the convulsions until professional assistance is available.

Prevention: During lactation feed lots of milk and bone meal to the bitch. Your vet will advise quantities. (See also Unconsciousness; Obstetrics; Diet for Brood Bitch; Analgesics; Convulsions.)

Miscarriage or Abortion

Miscarriages are infrequent among bitches, but they do occur as the result of an infection, a hormonal imbalance, an accident, or poor feeding. The fetus is expelled from the uterus before the end of the normal gestation period, which is fifty-eight to sixty-three days.

Early symptoms: As the birth process begins, the pregnant bitch will show signs of discomfort and restlessness, accompanied by bleeding from the vulva. This bleeding is followed by a clear discharge from the vulva. Then the miscarriage takes place, usually quite rapidly and painlessly, since the embryos are soft and small.

Emergencies: In rare instances, severe hemorrhage occurs during the birth or immediately afterward.

Treatment: Try to stanch the bleeding by applying an absorbent cotton pad to the vagina. If the free flow of blood is prevented, blood pressure inside the uterus should rise, causing the blood to clot and reducing the danger of hemorrhaging. Keep the animal calm and quiet. Get professional help without delay.

In extreme cases, when no vet is available and the bitch is hemorrhaging very badly, insert a roll of sterile gauze, a bit at a time, into the animal's vagina. Use your fingers. Make sure that you leave a tag end of the roll dangling, so that it can be removed later. Because of danger from infection, this is definitely a last resort.

Mismating

If a bitch mates with an undesirable dog, take her to a

veterinarian within thirty-six hours. An injection of di-ethylstilbestrol will nullify the conception.

Warning: Never attempt to force mating dogs apart. This could cause severe pain and hemorrhage in both ani-mals. It is also a wasted effort, since conception usually occurs within two to three minutes of penetration.

Mother Dog Eating Her Puppies

A bitch having her first litter should be carefully watched, for in certain instances she may attempt to eat her young. This is not as monstrous nor as abnormal as it sounds.

Causes: It may be the result of a natural fright response, but more often it is caused by a faulty placenta-eating instinct. In this case, the mother simply does not know where the placenta (afterbirth) ends and her newborn puppies begin.

Prevention: If a bitch seems nervous or overprotective toward her newborn litter, or if she objects to strangers (or even family) handling her young, humor her. Keep the strangers and the rest of the family away from the pups.

Of course, children are the main offenders and it is difficult to refuse them the delights of handling newborn puppies, but if the puppies' mother shows any resentment, this must be done. After all, they are *her* puppies.

Nipple Soreness

Cause: This condition is often seen while the female is nursing her litter. It is caused by the nails of the puppies pricking the soft flesh of the mother's teats.

Symptoms: The puppies will be screaming for food. The bitch's nipples will be red and cracked.

Treatment: If the mother's nipples are sore and red, apply lanolin or Vaseline ® twice a day. If Vaseline ® is used, make certain that it is rubbed in well. Wipe off the excess with absorbent cotton.

If the nipples have become cracked, bathe them three times a day in a solution made from ½ teaspoon boric acid added to 1 cup water. After bathing, dry the nipples gently but thoroughly with cotton and apply lanolin or Vaseline ®.

Prevention: The nails of puppies should be filed once a week.

Obstetrics

Generally, birth occurs fifty-eight to sixty-three days after conception, though a bitch may give birth a week early or a week late.

Signs of approaching birth: About six hours before birth, the mother becomes restless and begins preparing a place to have her litter (usually the most inconvenient place). Vomiting may occur. The animal's body temperature drops to about 98° F., a day before she is due. The vulva becomes enlarged and pinkish. The pelvic ligaments slacken, causing some loss of coordination of the hind legs.

Stages of labor: An hour or so before birth, the mother grows increasingly nervous, and may start glancing at her flanks. There are occasional contractions of the abdomen —one every ten minutes, becoming more frequent. The bitch may lie down as the contractions become more frequent. As the fetus enters the pelvis, there is definite straining. The water bag, which looks like a black grape, appears at the vulva. The mother will lick the water bag to rupture it. Several minutes or a few hours after the water breaks, the puppies, each in its own sac, begin to appear. Sometimes the nose and feet of the puppy protrude from the vulva. More often the entire puppy in its sac is expelled. If the bitch continues to strain and birth does not occur, a vet should be called. Often the mother will help as the puppy's head comes through.

Complications: If there is more than a two-minute delay after the head and front legs are out, the puppy should be gently pulled out. Use a towel to grip without slipping. Grip as high as you can. It is essential that the puppy be extracted as quickly and as carefully as possible.

Some puppies are born head first, some are born tail first. Both positions are normal, but if the puppy is born tail first, it should come out fairly rapidly. After the water bag has broken, the puppy should be out within five to ten minutes. If the puppy is not out in ten minutes, telephone a vet.

If the puppy is born with the membranous sac surrounding it still intact, and if the mother is preoccupied with another part of the birth process and neglects to remove the sac, remove it yourself rapidly. Every puppy should be checked immediately to be sure its mouth is free of mucus, enabling it to breathe freely. If breathing does not occur at once, rub the puppy briskly with a soft bath towel. If this does not work, hold the puppy in your hand, nesting its back in your palm, and swing it in a downward arc, stopping abruptly at the bottom of the arc. This can loosen mucus obstructing the throat; or try mouth-to-mouth respiration. Do not give up for at least twenty minutes. Once breathing has begun, put the puppy back with its mother and let her lick it dry.

Umbilical cord: The bitch should bite through the umbilical cord after each puppy comes out of the sac. If the cord is not cut, tie it off with clean, boiled sewing thread, two inches from the puppy, and cut it off on the side of the knot farthest away from the pup.

Afterbirth: After all the puppies are born, more membranes may be expelled. A greenish discharge from the bitch's vagina several hours after giving birth is quite normal.

Postpuerperal Metritis

This condition causes an abnormal vaginal discharge shortly after the bitch has given birth.

Symptoms: Excessive thirst; high fever; lethargy; depression. There is a heavy, dark, bloody discharge from the vagina two to five days after giving birth. This should not be confused with the slight, greenish brown discharge which is normal after a bitch has had a litter. The normal discharge is not accompanied by fever and greatly increased thirst.

Treatment: The above symptoms merit the immediate attention of a veterinarian.

Pyometritis (Pyometra)

This condition is usually seen in older (five to six years old) females, especially those that have irregular heat periods.

Cause: A pus-producing, abnormal development of the cells lining the womb. The condition occurs in two forms.

Open form: Creamy, foul-smelling vaginal discharge;

loss of appetite; increased thirst; vomiting; abdominal swelling. The condition is often confused with an abnormal heat period. However, pyometra is not an infectious disease, so there will not be any dramatic rise in body temperature.

Closed form: There is no visible sign of a discharge because the bitch's cervix remains closed and the uterus gradually fills up with pus. This produces a pronounced swelling of the abdomen, extreme lethargy, and increased thirst.

Treatment: Both forms of pyometritis are serious and require surgical treatment. Consult a vet immediately.

12

Poisoning

Poisoning: General

Before proceeding to more detailed information regarding symptoms and treatments for common poisons, do please realize that in most instances it is not possible for the dog owner to accurately diagnose a specific poison from observation of symptoms alone. The only exception is when the owner has actually seen the dog eating a particular poison. In the majority of cases, treatment must be limited to the general procedure covering all forms of poisoning.

Symptoms: Vomiting; diarrhea; internal hemorrhage; incoordination; twitching; convulsions; coma; unconsciousness.

Treatment: The above symptoms are also present in many other conditions. Without additional evidence, it is difficult to be certain that they are caused by poison. However, if there are grounds to suspect that a dog has eaten a poison, and if the dog is conscious, make it vomit as soon as possible, unless a corrosive poison such as an acid or alkali is suspected.

When acids or corrosive poisons have been ingested,

vomiting is not desirable. When these poisons are suspected, give olive oil orally, up to one pint for very large dogs, and proportionately less for smaller dogs.

Subsequent treatment consists of administering the proper antidote (providing you can identify the poison) and treating any symptoms as they arise. Otherwise, administer what is known as the "universal antidote."

If possible, always bring a sample of the suspected poison and a sample of the dog's vomit to the vet along with the patient. If the poison can be determined quickly, much valuable time can be saved.

Technique for inducing vomiting: The simplest and fastest way to induce vomiting is to throw ordinary table salt into the back of its mouth. (See How to Open a Dog's Mouth.) The quantity of table salt will vary depending upon the dog's size: one tablespoon salt for smaller dogs, three tablespoons for large dogs.

Universal Antidote: When the type of poison is not known, administer a universal antidote, consisting of: 2 parts charcoal (burned toast), 1 part magnesium oxide (milk of magnesia), 1 part tannic acid (strong tea). Give one tablespoon of this mixture per 20 pounds body weight. (See Force Feeding.)

If the dog is unconscious: Do not induce vomiting. Get it to a vet. Make sure the tongue is hanging out. Prop open the dog's jaw with an empty matchbox or spool.

If the dog has been in physical contact with toxic or corrosive substances: Wash the affected area clean with liberal amounts of clean water. Do not use soap.

If the dog is hyperexcited or having convulsions: Protect the animal from hurting itself by following the procedure for fits and convulsions. (See Fits.)

If there is poison on the skin: If a poison has contacted the skin or hair, bathe the affected portions with soap and water. Even if the poison does not burn the skin, it must be removed immediately, otherwise the dog will lick its coat and ingest the poison.

Acid and Alkali Poisons

Common acid poisons: Sulfuric acid (found in defoliants); car batteries; nitric acid; hydrochloric acid (drain cleaners).

Symptoms: Inflamed patches on the skin. When the dog licks them, this leads to: burning of the mouth, demonstrated by the dog's pawing violently at its mouth and by profuse dribbling of saliva; vomiting. Get professional help.

Treatment for acid poisoning: Administer up to 6 tablespoons of a solution made by adding 2 tablespoons sodium bicarbonate to 1 pint water. Force-feed egg whites and milk. Then force-feed up to one pint olive oil for very large dogs and proportionately less for smaller animals. Get the animal to the vet.

Treatment for acid burns: Bathe the inflamed patches with a solution of 4 tablespoons sodium bicarbonate to 1 pint water.

Common alkali poisons: Caustic soda; caustic potash; very large amounts of sodium bicarbonate and sodium carbonate.

Treatment for alkali poisons: Give 2 tablespoons of a solution made by adding 2 tablespoons of vinegar to 1 pint water. Wash the mouth out with vinegar. Then get professional help.

Treatment for alkali burns on the skin: Apply vinegar to alkali burns by pouring it directly over the burn, or by saturating a rag with vinegar and applying the rag to the burn. Then get professional help.

Warning: Do not administer emetics or attempt to induce vomiting.

Arsenic Poisoning

Sources: Rat and mouse poisons; ant poisons; insecticides; sheep and cattle dips; chemicals often found around smelting works and mines. Arsenic is also a common impurity found in many chemicals.

Symptoms: Acute arsenic poisoning may lead to death so quickly that there is no time to observe symptoms. Call a vet. Smaller doses of arsenic produce symptoms which include: intense abdominal pain; vomiting; staggering; diarrhea; collapse; coma; death. The breath of a dog suffering from arsenic poisoning will have a strong smell of garlic.

Treatment: If the animal is conscious, induce vomiting. Force-feed the dog a solution made by adding 2 tablespoons bicarbonate of soda to 1 pint water. Give the animal an enema of warm soapy water. Administer demulcents—substances that cover the irritated stomach lining—such as milk, or glycerin and water. (See Poisoning: General; Enema.)

Insulin Poisoning (Accidental Overdose)

Cause: Diabetic dogs receiving insulin treatment at home may be inadvertently overdosed, causing the dog to stagger and finally collapse. This usually occurs within an hour after treatment.

Symptoms: These vary from staggering and incoordination to unconsciousness.

Treatment: If the dog is still conscious, give one-half teaspoon of powdered sugar for small dogs, up to five teaspoons for large dogs. If the dog has lost consciousness, and a vet is not immediately available, mix sugar and water in the amounts given above. Pour a little at a time into the dog's mouth. Take great care not to choke the unconscious dog with the sugar water. Hold the dog upright. (See Force-Feeding.)

Mercury Poisoning

Sources: Antiseptics and fungicides, broken thermometers and barometers.

Symptoms: Early symptoms are vomiting and diarrhea. If death does not occur immediately from shock, the early symptoms are followed by ulceration of the mouth and tongue, then acute kidney failure.

Treatment: The absorption of mercury into the system is very rapid, and swift treatment is essential. If the dog's stomach can be emptied within half an hour of ingestion, there is a good chance of recovery.

Induce vomiting by throwing a tablespoon of salt into

the back of the dog's mouth. (See How to Open a Dog's Mouth.) The dog should then be force-fed raw egg whites and milk (2 egg whites to ½ pint milk). At the side of the dog's mouth, the lips form a pouch. Pull the pouch out a little and spoon a bit of the egg white and milk into the pouch. Tip the dog's head back slightly, and the dog will swallow. Repeat. Then induce vomiting again.

Phosphorus Poisoning

Sources: Red matches; rat and mouse poisons; roach poisons; the striking surfaces of matchboxes; fireworks.

Symptoms: The classic symptoms of staggering, abdominal pain, and vomiting are present. In phosphorus poisoning the vomit will glow in the dark. The dog's breath and vomit will have a strong odor of garlic. Following the onset of these symptoms, there is a period of apparent recovery that may last from three to four hours to several days. When this recovery period ends, abdominal pain and vomiting recur together with jaundice (a yellowish tinge appears in the eyes and mucous membranes) and there are nervous symptoms which, if ignored, will lead to coma and death.

Treatment: Treatment must not be delayed. At the first suspicion of phosphorus poisoning, induce vomiting by throwing a spoonful of salt into the back of the dog's mouth.

The specific antidote for phosphorus poisoning is given below but if these chemicals are not immediately available, administer the universal antidote instead. (See Poisoning: General.)

After causing the dog to vomit, force-feed a solution of 1 teaspoon of 1% copper sulfate to 1 pint water. Induce vomiting again. Then force-feed a solution of 1 teaspoon potassium permanganate (available at drugstores) to 1 pint water. (See Force-Feeding.) Give the dog an enema of warm, soapy water. (See Enemas.)

Do not feed the dog any fats for the next five days. (See Diet.)

Sedative Overdose

Sedatives, in the form of sleeping pills, are often left around by careless owners and eaten by unwary pets.

Symptoms: The dog will stagger about and appear very drowsy. It will keep trying to go to sleep. There may not be an empty pill container to confirm your suspicions. The dog may have eaten it along with the pills.

Treatment: Contact a vet. Induce vomiting. Administer stimulants. Strong tea or black coffee, cooled, should also be given.

Keep the dog awake. Walk or drag the dog around if necessary. Keep the animal walking until the effects wear off. If the dog keeps falling asleep, slap its face to keep it awake.

Strychnine Poisoning

Sources: Rat, mouse, and mole poisons.

Symptoms: The first symptoms of strychnine poisoning are excessive nervousness, restlessness, noticeable twitching of the muscles, and stiffness of the neck. As the condition progresses, these symptoms become more pronounced and convulsions suddenly occur. In convulsions caused by strychnine poisoning, the limbs are extended and the neck is curved upwards and backwards.

During the early stages, these convulsions are sporadic, but they become progressively more frequent until any external stimulus—the slightest noise or touch, even a current of air—will produce them. During this later stage, the pupils are widely dilated, covering nearly the whole surface of the eyeballs. Finally, death is caused by the inability to breathe, due to paralysis of the respiratory muscles.

Treatment: If the dog is having convulsions, it must be anesthetized by a vet. Do not try to take the dog to the vet. You will not make it. Have the vet come to the dog.

If convulsions have not yet begun, induce vomiting. Then force-feed the dog up to a pint of strong cold tea (tannic acid). Further treatment must be left to the vet.

While waiting for the vet, it is important to keep the dog very quiet and insulated from any external stimuli which may trigger convulsions. Place the dog in a quiet, darkened room.

Index